DEAD MAN TO IRONMAN

DEAD MAN TO IRONMAN

A TEN MONTH JOURNEY FROM DEAD MEAT TO ATHLETE

PAUL SMITH

pitch

First published by Pitch Publishing, 2020

Pitch Publishing
A2 Yeoman Gate
Yeoman Way
Worthing
Sussex
BN13 3QZ
www.pitchpublishing.co.uk
info@pitchpublishing.co.uk

A CIP catalogue record is available for this book from the British Library.

ISBN 978 1 78531 617 3

Typesetting and origination by Pitch Publishing

Printed and bound in India by Replika Press Pvt. Ltd.

Contents

Foreword 9
The Long Road to Diagnosis. 13
My Appendix – Take One 23
My Appendix – Take Two 36
Diagnosis Day 46
Seeing your Parents Can Be a Real Pain 55
Making Sense of the Big C. 60
Keep Calm and Swim 66
Kicking off a Ten-Week Block 75
In the Presence of Ironmen. 87
Moviprep and the Snake of Doom 100
Pseudo Mix What? 109
The Race for Life. 116
The Mother of all Surgery 132
Wakey Wakey .141
Chemo Haze, All in My Brain 151
A Dirty Protest and Drain Number Three. 160
Fifty Shades of Green 171
Just a Little Prick Sir 179
Home Sweet Home. 191
Slow and Steady 199
The Long Course Weekend – Part 1. 215
The Long Course Weekend – Part 2. 226
The Long Course Weekend – Part 3. 237
The Highs and Lows of the Long Distance Triathlete 245
The Final Push 260
Swim 271
Bike 285
Run 299
Epilogue 310
Acknowledgements 316

for Maria

Foreword

YOU'RE 43, happily cruising through life and you've just been diagnosed with cancer.

When your life suddenly turns upside down like that, what are you going to do next? When I asked myself that question I decided it would be a good idea to do an Ironman triathlon.

That improbable seed was sown way back in 2013 during a particularly slow day at work when my good friend Tom boldly stated that he was going to do an Ironman 70.3 in Mallorca the following summer. I almost spat out my tea in disbelief. An Ironman 70.3 is a middle-distance triathlon, or, more precisely, a 1.2-mile swim, followed by a 56-mile bike ride and a half marathon.

When I eventually stopped laughing I realised that I was actually quite inspired by the revelation: he wasn't exactly the athletic type and it seemed like a ridiculously difficult feat of endurance. That winter I watched on with interest as he knuckled down and trained through some truly miserable winter mornings, and, although I would never tell him to his face, I was quietly impressed and the endless talk about it all wasted many long days at work when work was the last thing either of us could be bothered with.

The following summer the Ironman 70.3 Mallorca was duly completed, and the pasty, slightly obese man who walked out of the door just a week before returned a triumphant tanned and toned athlete with a great-looking medal to prove it. My congratulations and interest quickly dried up, however, as I didn't hear the end of it. He would spend the whole day droning on about his new-found sporting prowess whilst sipping tea from his Ironman mug and taking big manly gulps from his Ironman-branded water bottle.

We both ran a bit and enjoyed riding our bikes but I could no longer hold a flame to the newly discovered athlete that now sat opposite me. I was secretly a bit jealous, but in equal measure I was mightily impressed.

There was one big issue taking the shine off of it for him though; this fantastic achievement was never really going to be good enough. His big brother was a veteran of several full long-distance Ironman triathlons and this fact ensured that there were no bragging rights at home. Little brother was only half of an Ironman after all, so the talk in the office turned to completing a full Ironman race, which is a long-distance triathlon consisting of a 2.4-mile swim followed by a 112-mile bike ride and then a full marathon, absolutely ridiculous mind-bending numbers. I thought to myself, could I manage that? No fucking chance.

The biggest problem I have is that at heart I'm a self-confessed lazy bastard, I always have been. I talk a good game, buy all the kit and then fade away quietly until the next big thing comes along. I've dabbled in lots of sports and not really mastered any. My strength, if I have one, is that I love to be outdoors and I love to ride my bikes, surf and walk in the mountains. I have a degree of grit and stamina when I need it but focus has never really been my strong point. The bottom line is I'm a cruiser. So could I break that habit and channel enough desire and determination to achieve something like an Ironman?

Who knows? But the famous red tattoo that many Ironman finishers wear would look very cool. There I go again, all about the show with little regard for any substance.

In my favour, as I've got older, I have discovered a more adventurous streak that pushes me a little more. I completed a couple of half-marathons which, even five years before, would have been simply unheard of, so maybe the inner athlete was stirring in me after all. All this talk of being an Ironman was getting infectious.

I had already upped my exercise regimes following the lead set by my new sporting mentor and had for a while intended to seriously 'think' about doing a triathlon. I was definitely a self-confessed MAMIL (middle-aged man in lycra) and I was bitten by the British Tour de France successes like most of the mid-life crisis bracket males in the country. I was swimming for the first time and I was even out jogging on a regular basis; in fact, I'd never been so motivated to buy new kit in all my life.

The downside to all this enthusiasm was that I was already finding the training tough, especially the running, which was becoming a real problem for me. In previous sporadic bouts of exercise I always managed to increase my distance and speed quite quickly, but this time it was a struggle. My lungs would be bursting after a couple of miles and my shuffling running style was positively geriatric. I could only put it down to old age so I gamely carried on.

I was following the start of an Ironman training programme as a taster and as it was being dissected in detail every day at work, I couldn't give up at this early stage. How on earth was my germinating seed of completing an Ironman going to grow into a mighty oak if I couldn't even muster the energy to run around the block a few times?

Little did I know it then, but that was soon going to be the least of my worries.

The Long Road to Diagnosis

THE ROAD to a cancer diagnosis is often a long one and can be full of missed opportunities and regrets. The first time I really felt that anything was wrong with me was back in early 2013 when I started having sporadic bouts of stomach ache. I wasn't truly diagnosed until September 2014 when I went to the North Hampshire Hospital in Basingstoke for the first time and saw the excellent Mr Mohamed. That was about 14 months after it started, but in truth my symptoms probably started long before that.

For as long as I can remember, I would occasionally develop a cramping aching sensation in my lower right abdomen. It was never enough to drag me to the doctor but it was always enough to make me feel a bit unwell and lose my appetite. It would strike every couple of months and last about three or four days until it would subside again. I self-diagnosed myself from the internet with all sorts of random ailments from irritable bowel syndrome to old age, so I didn't think too much of it.

Over time the bouts slowly started to get more serious and in March 2014 I took my first sick days off work as a result of it. I had developed a shivery fever and a temperature this time around, and as I was feeling pretty run-down I took the Thursday and Friday off to recover. As usual I was fighting fit within a couple of days so was back to work the following Monday.

I had another attack in April; this time it came with less of a gap between occurrences but wasn't quite as severe. I sat at work huffing and puffing, feeling tired and very out of sorts. I mentioned to my colleagues that I wasn't feeling well again and was roundly told to get a grip of myself and man up.

I took their advice and soldiered on, but by now I was thinking that I would need to see a doctor and discuss it. Now, I had self-diagnosed it as gallstones, grumbling appendix and IBS, but being generally of good health I knew that something wasn't right.

I'm a two-day-a-year, if that, type of sick note. I just don't do sick, but that calendar year I was on my sixth day already and there were countless more that I hadn't taken off which maybe I should have, all down to this mystery illness.

It was May when Tom had gone off to Mallorca for his Ironman 70.3. He travelled with family and friends for a week's holiday and several of them were going to do the event. We had talked endlessly at work about his training programme and although work had been busy and he had missed a few crucial late training sessions as a result, he appeared to be as ready as he would ever be.

In contrast, my sniffs at a training plan had been sporadic to say the least – constant bouts of illness and fatigue had put paid to each attempt I had made to get myself going. The training plan we were following was the Don Fink *Be Iron Fit* programme. It's a structured plan with progressive increments in all three disciplines of swimming, running and cycling to bring you up to the standard of fitness required to complete an Ironman. Two-thirds through the programme was the middle-distance preparation race and this was the point that Tom had trained up to.

The programme is split into three different levels. Just Finish, Intermediate and Advanced; they all follow the same pattern but with different intensities. Tom's brother and his partner had used it to good effect to complete Ironman Zurich and Sweden previously, so we knew it worked. We would train using the Just Finish programme, which aimed to complete the race in between 15 and 17 hours.

Talks were in their early stages regarding completing an Ironman ourselves, but the seed was now sown and we were both nibbling around the edges and sounding out what was really required to go the distance.

On the day of the race I kept an eye on the results as they came in online and could see that Tom had finished in six hours and 54 minutes, a fantastic achievement. I was really impressed and so pleased for him. I couldn't wait till he got back and we could dissect all the gory details.

When he returned to work he looked very well, tanned and even a bit slimmer with an impressive medal to show for his efforts. He had his shiny Ironman mug which he was insisting I fill with tea every five minutes, seeing as I was now very clearly his inferior.

At first he was very understated. 'How did it go?' I'd ask.

'Yeah, it was good mate,' was the nonchalant response, but the more I probed him the clearer it became that it was no walk in the park.

His first fear had been that the sea swim would be non-wetsuit – if the temperature rises to 25 degrees Celsius, the swim is deemed to be too warm for wetsuits so then only swimsuits are allowed. The thing with a wetsuit is that it gives you buoyancy. This has two benefits: it allows you to float in the water and not drown when you are tired, and it keeps you flatter in the water and allows you to swim more easily without using your legs to keep you up in the water. This saves a lot of energy and without a wetsuit a swim of 1,900 metres is a long way for a novice and a daunting prospect, especially in the sea. Tom was saved from a drowning on the morning of the race by the thin margin of only one and a half degrees Celsius.

The 90 kilometre (56 mile) bike leg starts with a long, hard climb out of town into the Tramuntana Mountains, followed by an equally long, fast descent and a quick ride back into the transition area. By his own account he nailed it, overtaking people both on the climb and the descent and then rolling smoothly back into town, at speed, for the run.

That's when it all started to unravel – the run was a straight out-and-back half-marathon along the promenade and coast road. A blisteringly hot and dry run under a cloudless sky with no shade from the 30-degree heat anywhere. It quickly turned into a dehydrated horror show of dripping sweat and never-ending shuffling that wasn't helped by his father, who was sat in a shady roadside bar shouting ever more irritating encouragement with a cold beer in his hand.

But it got done and I could see how pleased he was. This was a real sporting achievement – there was no hiding on that course and you either did it or did not. He did, and I was thinking, 'You know what? I want some of that.' I would just need to man up as recommended by my work colleagues and get down to it.

June came around and it was a hot one, our antiquated office had no air conditioning and was roasting us alive. It was a sauna in there and to cap it all off, I was sore again. I felt exhausted all day and was so hot at night I'd wake up drenched in sweat. One night the bed was soaked so badly we had to change the sheets at three in the morning.

That week at work went very slowly. I just couldn't get myself going, but eventually it was Friday and the whole office were out on the town for a colleague's leaving drinks as he was off to a new department.

It's a good time to say that I am a police detective by trade, so these events always followed the same well-trodden boozy path. A lunchtime start in a pub and then on for a curry or even more drinks if it was deemed by the committee on the day that eating was cheating and was going to be an unnecessary distraction.

We had gathered in a very pleasant shady pub garden by the river at about two in the afternoon. It was a lovely sunny day and was the perfect place to kick off a drunken evening's entertainment, but as I sat nursing my first pint I just wasn't feeling it, the beer tasted sour and I just couldn't get it down. Anyone who knows me will tell you that this is very unusual, I do like a beer. The next round arrived and I made the cardinal sin of asking for a shandy. I knew the abuse that was coming but I couldn't face another straight pint. This alone should have been enough proof of how unwell I was becoming. I made it until about 6:30pm, when I made my excuses as the group were moving on to a curry house. I was a sweaty mess and I felt terrible. My friends joked about how much of a lightweight I was and I wandered back to the train station. I went back home and straight into bed by 8:30.

If I'd only realised then that developing a serious bout of sepsis was lightweight, I may have made the effort to stay out a bit later.

The next day I felt no better and we had to cancel a dinner party with some of our neighbours which had been planned for weeks. My wife Maria took them the foil-wrapped dinner she had prepared for them to have at theirs and I was back in bed by 8pm again.

Reading this it would be easy to say, 'What an idiot, its bloody obvious that you weren't well, why didn't you go to the doctor?'

Well you would be dead right and this time I did. I said to myself if I'm not better by Monday morning I'll go to the doctor. In the time-honoured tradition of men worldwide who are considering a trip to the doctors, I obviously woke up Monday morning feeling much better, but I did still feel as if I had a bit of a temperature and four days of feeling rough told me I wasn't well, so my day was now mapped out for me.

I was straight up and out of the door at 7:30am because, as with the sorry state of all doctors' surgeries these days, you can really struggle to get an appointment. You have to call up on the day for an emergency appointment and planned appointments are booked for at least three weeks in the future. The phone lines open at 8am and one second after eight they become permanently engaged with no call-back or queueing functions, so you hang up and ring again and again and again. Forty minutes later, if you haven't already succumbed to your ailments, you might eventually get through when, surprise surprise, no appointments are left for that day.

To avoid disappointment the best thing to do is physically drag your sickly body to the front counter at 8am on the dot, so that's what I did. As I drove past the surgery at 7:45am, I could see at least ten people in a dishevelled line outside the door. I parked and obediently took my place in the coughing and hacking line of misery snaking around the building. I reckoned I was number 12 by then as another couple of pensioners had snuck up before I had time to park the car and run back up the road. By 8am, when the doors were ceremonially opened to an ironic cheer from someone further forward in the line, at least six more had joined the party.

We shuffled forward and took our turn to make our demands of the already over-stressed receptionist. It was 8:10am when I got my appointment for 9:30am, so, already pleased with my day's work, I went home, put my feet up and downed a boiling hot cup of tea before heading straight back out of the door for my appointment. Sitting in the doctors' waiting area, I wondered if I could even feel the pain any more and pressed my fingers into my side hoping to bring it on a bit so the doctor didn't think I was a complete hypochondriac. If the worst it had been in the preceding week was a six out of ten, then today it was only a two, and a two was definitely wasting the doctor's time in my book but I was there so I resolved to see what they had to say.

I was called through and took my place in the customary plastic chair next to his desk as I explained my symptoms. I told him that I had researched it on the internet and thought I had gallstones. He agreed that it sounded very much like it and asked me to lie on the bed so he could examine me.

I pulled up my top, unzipped my jeans, lowering them to my hips, and lay back staring at the ceiling as he gently but firmly felt his way around my abdomen.

'Does it hurt here?'

'No.'

'How about here?'

'No.'

'Here?'

'Yes, a little bit.'

'Ok, how about here?'

'No.'

'If you can just hang on for a moment I'm going to pop out and fetch one of my colleagues.'

Despite the calm in his voice, my head popped straight up from the pillow to look at him as he said, 'I won't be a second.' I watched the back of him scoot out of the door and my very first thought was that it was a good job I came down as there must be something wrong with me after all. I lay back and continued looking at the dog-eared poster of a Bavarian castle that had been taped to the ceiling whilst I waited.

He stepped back into the room with another doctor in tow, whom I recognised from the surgery. The second doctor then got hands on.

'Can you feel that?' asked the first.

'Yes, yes I can,' affirmed the second.

They shared a few knowing glances and nods between themselves and the second doctor said cryptically, 'I would. Yes. Definitely.' It was clear that they had discussed something out of my earshot before returning to the room.

The second doctor left the room and the first told me to get dressed as he returned to his desk. I was starting to feel a bit nervous as I parked myself back in the plastic chair next to him.

As he typed he turned to me and said, 'I don't want you to worry, it may be nothing, but I'm going to refer you to the hospital right now. I can feel a mass near to your appendix and I'd like the hospital to take a look at it today.' Today! Bloody hell, how serious is it, I wondered. 'Try not to worry too much as it might not be anything serious but I'd like the hospital to look at it.

'Go home and I will make some phone calls and type a referral letter which you can pick up on your way to the hospital. Will you have any problems getting to the hospital?'

'No,' I said, 'I'll call the wife.' So off home I went. Thirty minutes later the phone went and the doctor said, 'I've made arrangements, can you get to the ultrasound department in an hour? Please pop back to the surgery and pick up your referral letter on the way. You can read it if you like but there really is no need. If you do read it, try not to panic.'

Oh, ok then.

I called work and told them I wouldn't be in as I was going to hospital but I promised I would man up and return to work as soon as possible.

My wife Maria rushed home from work and we hot-footed it straight down to the local hospital. Within the hour I was sat with her in the waiting area of the ultrasound on another uncomfortable plastic chair, with both of us wondering what to make of it all. I had no idea that this would turn into a week in hospital and my first painful experiences at the hands of the consultants.

My Appendix – Take One

THE FIRST thing I had to do when we arrived at the hospital was take myself straight down to phlebotomy, show the receptionist my letter and give up some blood samples for analysis. There must have been 30 people in the waiting area, but with the red sticker on my letter I was sent straight to the front of the queue and into the nurse's chair.

The nurses who work in this department all day are very skilled in taking blood, and before I knew it the 'gentle scratch' had filled at least four separate little phials which were whisked away through another door for fast-time analysis.

I've had injections before and had given blood previously so I have no real aversion to needles, but of course it's always unpleasant. It was something I would have to quickly start getting very used to. Within a matter of minutes I was out of phlebotomy with the customary cotton wool ball taped to my arm and following the coloured signs around the hospital corridors to the ultrasound.

As everything was happening so quickly, I didn't really have time to worry about what I was doing there, I had no idea what I was being tested for. The thought of cancer had risen in the back of my mind but it was more likely to be an appendicitis, so I wasn't going to worry. I was more relieved that I'd made the right decision to go to the doctor, as something clearly wasn't right in there.

I sat with Maria in the waiting area of the ultrasound department in the company of about three or four other people and waited. As an emergency drop-in, it was clear that I was going to have to wait for a bit to see someone as the schedule was already full.

We were told that we would need to wait for about an hour to be seen but I was pleased to be called forward in much less time than that by a consultant who poked his head out of a darkened side room and ushered us in.

He was every bit the eccentric doctor that you might see on the television. He was very well spoken, wearing a red cravat and sporting an equally red nose and cheeks, the perfect caricature of an old army colonel. It was equally clear that he ran his department like the military and was quite sharp with the nurses and other assistants who were rushing to clear the backlog before their lunch break, one which I was contributing to.

Once inside the examination room he was instantly a lot calmer and personable as he explained to me that he would conduct an ultrasound examination as a mass had been detected on the side of my bowel by my doctor. I lifted my t-shirt and lowered my jeans and he applied some jelly to my abdomen as he pressed his ultrasound device firmly into my side and began moving it in gentle swirling motions.

The monitor was facing us but I couldn't make out anything distinctive on the screen. The only ultrasound images I had ever seen were when friends suddenly became grainy images of foetuses on their Facebook profiles, and I certainly hoped one of those wouldn't pop up on the screen. The colonel pointed out a darkened area in my right lower abdomen and said that he could see and feel the mass as described by the doctor. I was dressing when he told me I would be sent for an emergency scan to examine the area further and I would need to remain on the hospital grounds while it was arranged.

He explained to us that it could be several things including an inflamed appendix, but this was also the first time that the word cancer came up – it could also be a tumour, which could indicate cancer. I was told to try not to worry at this stage as it could be many things but it did require further urgent investigation.

He could tell I still had a temperature and said that he would make arrangements for me to be admitted. He asked us to stay in the ultrasound department while he went off to secure me a bed for the night. It was all starting to get a bit more serious now, but I was actually feeling a lot better in myself and still felt a bit of a fraud. I just couldn't get my head around how ill I might have become.

The colonel returned and told me that we needed to move to the accident and emergency department as a gateway into the hospital. Half walking and half skipping behind him, we raced to keep up as he marched us double time through a giddying labyrinth of corridors.

It was packed in the accident and emergency waiting area and people were lying on trolley beds and sat on chairs in the corridor waiting to be moved on – it looked like a scene from a disaster movie. Some people looked like they were already dead and others looked like they shouldn't be there at all. One bored-looking child even had one of those big fat cartoon bandages on their thumb with a bow tied on the top of it.

The colonel introduced us to a young doctor who already appeared to have been briefed that I was coming, and I was sat in a chair and told to wait. The colonel said he would be back later to make sure that I was being taken care of and I thanked him as he marched off back down the corridor. I could hear him shouting loud instructions to some other poor sod as he disappeared out of sight.

I was now getting hot and sweaty again. The temperature in the hospital was really uncomfortable anyway but my fever was starting to kick back in and I had that sticky hangover-type of clamminess going on. As I was settling in for the long haul, one of the small private examination rooms opposite me became available. I wasn't expecting to be moved as there appeared to be other, more deserving patients lying on beds and groaning around me, but the doctor ushered me in and told me to lie on the bed and get comfortable.

In a few minutes he came back with two nurses and told me that my blood results were back and it was clear that I was fighting a serious blood infection. Apparently my white blood cell count was through the roof and he would need to put me on a drip of antibiotics straight away. A tray appeared with all the things he needed and within seconds there was a cannula in my left forearm and a clear drip bag hanging above my head, and I realised now that I probably did deserve my place in the queue after all.

The doctor then apologised as he told me he would also need to examine my prostate; if I would be more comfortable he could clear the room for it. I knew straight away that this involved a finger up my backside and I didn't relish the prospect of sticking my puckered bumhole in the air in front of two attractive young nurses, two junior doctors and my wife, so I told him I would be happier if I could just face the other way. He laughed and came around the other side of the bed as he stretched a rubber glove over his hand. I held my breath nervously waiting and it was all over in a second – I barely felt it. Apparently that bit of me was fine. All I had to do now was wait for my scan and a bed to become free in the main hospital.

My antibiotic drip was changed for another full bag and more bloods were taken. I must have been in that room for about three hours when I heard the colonel out in the corridor. I was sure he probably should have gone home by then. He came into my room and appeared genuinely annoyed that I was still lying in accident and emergency. He assured me that I would be moved on soon and off he went to remonstrate with someone about it. I didn't see him again but I often think back fondly of him. I'm convinced that he suspected that it was more than just appendicitis he had seen on the ultrasound and he really looked out for me that day.

A porter arrived and I was put into a wheelchair and whisked around to the CT scan department. Apparently I was now far too ill to walk there. I went straight through and was asked to get into one of those blue boil-washed hospital gowns and my drip was detached so I could lie on the scanner. I'd seen these on the television before, it was a big doughnut-shaped machine that you slide through on a moving bed. A little animated smiley face tells you to hold your breath and remain still at certain times as some sort of device spins around inside the doughnut at high speed firing dangerous laser beams, so that it can take a cross-sectional image of your body.

I remained in my gown and was wheeled straight up to the bowel ward where a bed was waiting for me. I have spent a lot of time in bowel wards over the past couple of years but the thing that hits you when you get wheeled in for the first time is the smell. I wonder what I was expecting? Maybe roses, it is the bowel ward after all. That sweet scent of medicated diarrhoea never leaves you. I can smell it now.

My bed was in a small ward of six patients with the usual curtains around them and I was parked up slap bang in the middle. All the beds appeared to be occupied by what looked like ancient mummies. They were all either asleep or dead, except for one who lifted his head, nodding an acknowledgement to me from across the room as I hopped up on to my bed and lay back down.

There was another round of blood tests and bag changes and my blood pressure and temperature were taken; throughout the day I had developed a roaring temperature and could now feel that I was really burning up. Maria had been home and brought me a couple of changes of clothes and a wash bag, along with my laptop, iPod and some magazines, so I had plenty to keep me occupied. She stayed with me for the rest of the evening before heading off home.

I sat on my bed wondering when someone might come and tell me what was going to happen next; I had missed the daily ward rounds so there were no more consultants until the next day. You soon get to know the ebb and flow of hospital life as you observe it from the comfort of your bed. The nurses are there to care for you but they don't have much medical information to share, similarly the junior ward doctors who are in attendance for the more serious stuff can't really act without the say-so of the consultants. This makes the long wait between the fleeting consultant visits even more frustrating if you have any questions like, 'Can you tell me what's wrong with me, maybe?'

A nurse appeared holding a bed pan and wide-eyed I prayed it wasn't meant for me. It was a relief to see her begin pulling the curtain around the bed next to me. I could hear the old boy straining and farting behind the thin piece of fabric dividing us, so I put my headphones on and listened to some heavy metal. Unfortunately the thin curtain couldn't protect my nostrils from everything that was occurring. Bloody hell, I think I will go for a little walk.

When I returned the lights had been dimmed and everyone was already asleep. I lay back on the bed just as a doctor stuck his head around the curtain. 'Mr Smith? Hi, I know it's late but I wanted to come and give you some good news, we've examined your scans and it's a particularly bad case of appendicitis. I know there has been some talk of cancer today [has there?!], so I wanted to pop up and reassure you so that you weren't up all night worrying about it.'

'Wow, thank you. That's great news. I appreciate it.'

'You are very welcome, the consultant will discuss options for treatment tomorrow,' and he was off. I lay on the bed taking it in. I had wondered if it was something more serious but this was great news. I texted Maria and turned in for the night. He needn't have worried about me not sleeping, that's for sure. The five elephants in the room rasping away in shifts throughout the night, alongside the fact that the lights were permanently on, machines beeped for hours before a nurse reset them, and the constant shouting of people with dementia mixed with the nurses crashing about outside put paid to any sleep I was planning on getting.

If you have ever been in hospital you will know just what an assault on the senses it is. Hospitals never sleep, just like most of their patients come to think of it. It's a wonder that anyone gets better in these places. It's like the shittiest hotel you've ever stayed in with really nice staff trying to make up for it. You doze all day and then stare at the ceiling all night.

The next morning the consultants made their rounds. It was almost comical as about ten people rushed in like the Keystone Cops behind the consultant and they all crowded around the bed trying to get a glimpse of me.

I was told that my appendix had likely been grumbling for some time and had enlarged and been encased in a fatty pocket, this is what could be felt and seen on the scans and was the body's way of protecting me from an infection. It had, however, now perforated and my blood tests indicated that I was developing sepsis. The priority would be to reduce the blood poisoning and the infection around the appendix before they could consider surgery. I would likely be in hospital until the end of the week and remain on the intravenous antibiotics until my blood results improved. To operate now would risk further dangerous infection and complications.

This made sense so I had no further questions for now. That morning someone had obviously taken pity on me so my bed, with me in it, was wheeled to a private room down the corridor. It was either that or I was now considered far too toxic to share a room with other sick people, but either way at least I would get some sleep that night.

Time goes by very slowly in hospital. You spend a lot of time staring around your room waiting for the next cup of tea, next blood test or your observations to be done. These little interludes really help to break up the day. You wait for your visiting times like a prisoner, and Maria came up to see me straight from work every day. My work colleagues helped keep me amused with non-stop abusive text messages telling me what a lazy git I was.

The next day the consultant decided to send me down for another ultrasound to see how the infection was getting on. So at about midday a porter arrived with a wheelchair, I hung my bag off the back and away we went.

The examination room I was wheeled into was a bit like a dentist's surgery with a reclining chair in the middle, bright lights on stalks with lots of machinery all around. The young doctor and an assisting nurse welcomed me in. The procedure was much like the colonel's but at the end of it the doctor turned to me and said, 'We could put a drain in that and see if we can get rid of some of the infection.'

It was the first I'd heard of this but I wasn't going to disagree if he thought it might help.

'We will need to give you a local anaesthetic and insert a needle into the appendix and then a tube to drain it off,' he continued. 'Are you ok with needles, it will be a bit uncomfortable?'

I signed a consent form and we were off, right there and then. I lay back on the dentist's chair as he prepared his equipment. Oh my god, what the hell is that! From the corner of my eye I got a glimpse of something that resembled a knitting needle with a massive syringe on the end of it. It was the type of thing you might shoot a whale with to sedate it. I took a deep breath as he hovered above me with it.

He explained that he would have to anaesthetise me in layers through the abdomen and I turned away as the needle slid into my side. I wasn't going to watch that. This was not the sharp scratch of an ordinary injection, it felt more like a sword or an arrow going into me. I took a sharp intake of breath and held it. Laying as stiff as a board, I felt the needle go in again and again, each time deeper and deeper. 'Ok, that's done.' I slumped back into the chair, let out my breath and uncurled my toes. I could feel the anaesthetic working so I relaxed. 'I now need to insert the drain, this bit might be more uncomfortable as I can't actually anaesthetise your bowel.'

I took another deep breath as he prepared. He had a tube the thickness of a pencil with the needle inside it in one hand and his ultrasound in the other so he could see what he was doing. I can't really explain what it feels like to have your bowels touched inside your body. It's a hideous, dull, radiating pain unlike anything that you will ever have experienced before. Pain is pain, right? Not really, this is very particular and I felt dizzy and sweaty. The nurse could see me gritting my teeth and as she took hold of my hand, I squeezed it hard.

The consultant was struggling to get the drain into the fatty mass around my appendix and needed three or four goes to be satisfied he was in. What felt like a lifetime later, he sat up with a contented look on his face and told me he was done.

He taped the tube in place and I could sit up. I was nauseous and giddy. Sweat was beading on my forehead and I could feel my back was soaked against the chair. I had pins and needles in my fingers and toes and my vision was closing in. I thought I was going to faint but the spit gathering in my mouth told me otherwise. 'I think I'm going to be sick.'

One of those grey cardboard party hats masquerading as a bowl that you get in hospital was thrust under my chin and I vomited. It was only liquid and I only vomited the once, but I instantly felt better. They gave me a couple of minutes to compose myself while they tidied up the room and clipped a bag on to the end of my drain. The porter was then called and came to wheel me back to my bed as a thin trickle of pink fluid started to drip down the tube.

As we rolled back along the corridor the porter asked me how it was. I was halfway through telling him how bad it was when I screamed out, 'BLOODY HELL, STOP!' I noticed out of the corner of my eye that the tube from the drain had got caught in the wheel of the wheelchair and was being dragged slowly away from me. Bloody hell that was a close call, I had visions of being dragged screaming over the front of the chair by my tube as it tore out leaving me lying under the wheels.

I gathered up my pipework and the rest of the journey back to my room was fortunately less eventful. As I lay back on my bed I reflected that at least I was in the game now – up until then I had still felt like I was a bit of a passenger on this ride – but after that procedure I could really justify my bed and status as a patient.

I remained in hospital until the Friday lunchtime with no further incidents of note other than when I caught the loop of my drain around the toilet door handle as I was coming out, that really made my eyes water I can tell you.

On the Friday morning the nurse came to remove my cannula and pull out the drain. I was a little apprehensive, as this was all done without any further anaesthetic. The nurse basically tugs on it till it's out. I lay back and held my breath again. It wasn't exactly painful but I could feel every inch of it sliding out of me. It really made me shudder and I swear I will never watch a movie in the same light when the hero gets shot or stabbed in the guts and carries on fighting or running around as normal, it's just not possible.

I was told prior to discharge that I would have to take two weeks' worth of strong antibiotics and would be seen back at the hospital in a month's time when an assessment would be made about further treatment.

Great, two weeks with my feet up. We had a cottage booked in Wales for the second week and the weather was looking good, so I would make the most of the time to get myself back up to strength. As we left the hospital that afternoon I reflected on how lucky I had been and how relieved I was to have made myself go to the doctor's that morning.

My Appendix – Take Two

I LEFT the hospital reasonably happy. I was feeling a lot better thanks to all the drugs that had been pumped into me, but I was very aware that it was still unfinished business as far as my appendix was concerned. My temperature was gone and all I had left to show for my time in hospital was a single stitch in the puncture wound which was busy dissolving under a plaster.

The second week came around quickly and we were off to North Wales. We were staying in a little cottage nestled in a beautiful cove on the Llyn Peninsula, right next to a fantastic pub on the beach, and the weather forecast was looking great. The lack of an afternoon drink to go with my antibiotics tormented me all week, but day by day I was slowly feeling more like my old self. One sunny afternoon we made some sandwiches and decided to go for a walk up the highest hill in the area. I walked up it like an old man and by the time we reached the top I was wheezing like I'd polished off 50

Marlboro Reds on the way up. I was completely done in and it was the first time I really understood how much had been taken out of me by that infection. My general fitness could only have been about 50 per cent.

Before I knew it, I was back at work for a week before my appointment at the hospital. It's easy to moan about the police as an employer, but you won't find a more understanding boss when you really need it. I was back and firing on all cylinders but I could feel the ache in my side sneaking back up on me. I wondered whether it was just the wounds healing from the drain that was inserted, but by the time of my appointment the following Monday the same old symptoms were rearing their ugly head again.

Maria travelled home to her parents in Slovakia that weekend for a visit which had been in the diary for a long time. She was worried about me going to the hospital on my own but I convinced her to go as I was sure nothing was likely to happen quickly.

That final weekend after waving Maria off, I was away in Yorkshire with Tom who was still living off his Ironman 70.3 success. We were in attendance for the grand depart of the Tour de France and were staying at the equally grandly titled Festival of Cycling at Harewood House near Leeds. We were very excited MAMILs as we were staying right at the start line and were very much looking forward to seeing all the top cycling stars.

'The historic start will roll through the grounds of the stately home in a carnival-like atmosphere,' said the brochure.

In truth it was shit. It pissed down with rain for pretty much the whole weekend and we stood around for hours to glimpse a few seconds of the pro cyclists riding past through the gaps in the heads of a five-deep crowd. We couldn't even get to see the official start as it was VIPs only and had been barricaded off from the rest of the general riff-raff like us, most of whom were wearing ridiculous-looking free cycling caps which had unceremoniously been flung from a passing float.

The festival of cycling itself consisted of a bouncy castle and some pointlessly cobbled-together stalls selling energy drinks and mountain bike accessories. There was what appeared to be a jumble sale of overpriced cycling clothing seconds and a small display of exotic £10,000 bicycles. The bar closed at 5pm, leaving about 1,500 people stuck in a muddy field in the rain with nothing to do.

The only entertainment was an outdoor cinema showing random cycling documentaries from the 1970s which didn't even have anything to do with the Tour de France. To add insult to injury, some poor buggers had to cycle on exercise bikes in the rain to generate the electricity to run it in some thinly veiled attempt by the organisers to claim some green credentials, or more likely to save money on electricity.

We were forced to hide from the rain in the gloom of our tent for most of the weekend, and in the first evening managed to drink our way through two boxes of warm rosé wine, which was all that was available from the crappy on-site shop. This poor choice of drink was forced upon us because we had already drunk all the beers we had brought with us out of sheer boredom earlier in the day. We spent most of the time drunkenly talking about doing an Ironman and what training and other events we could do to help with our preparation.

We ate endless barbecues as the mobile Morrisons supermarket lorry where we brought the wine from was selling packets of burgers and sausages for a pound each. The refrigerator in the lorry had broken down and they were offloading their stock before the ambient temperatures started to poison everybody. We reckoned some chancer had stolen a delivery lorry and was simply selling off its contents out of the back of it. To cap it all off, I had a front tyre blow-out in the fast lane of the motorway on the way home which nearly killed us both.

Despite the hangover and constipation from the three-day meat-and-wine fest, I knew I wasn't right again. The pains were back with a vengeance when I woke up on the Sunday morning, and I felt weak and sweaty by the time we got home; in truth, it felt like I was right back to square one.

I was at the hospital early for my appointment and I was in the outpatient department waiting with lots of other people of all ages and apparent ailments, and as usual I was the only one who looked like there was nothing wrong with me.

I was called forward right on time and went through to one of the examination rooms. I explained to the consultant that I was feeling a bit better but the pain had come back in my side. She examined me and straight away said she could feel the infection was growing again.

She explained that to operate would risk complications due to the excessive infection but she wanted to admit me today for an immediate appendectomy if I was in agreement, as it was clear that I wasn't improving as expected.

Today! Blimey, ok then. I was happy to hit it head on and get it done to be honest. I was told to go and give some blood samples first and, as I was on my own, to go home and pack a bag for at least three days in hospital. When I returned I was to come back to outpatients where I would be told which ward to report to. I needed to be back at the hospital in two hours if possible. 'Oh, and don't eat or drink anything either.'

When I returned from home, I was sent up to the same ward and the same private room I was in during my previous stay four weeks before. I was pleased to be in a private room again, remembering the circus going on down the corridor, and thought that I may be lucky and get some sleep this time around.

I had my vital signs and statistics taken by the nurses and got dressed into the hospital uniform of fetching washed-out blue gown and green compression stockings with my toes sticking out of the ends. I was wheeled back down for another scan and then sat waiting for the surgical consultants to come up and see me to discuss the operation. I had time to call Maria, who was ready to jump on a plane and come straight back home, but I managed to talk her out of it by promising to call her as soon as I could when I was out of surgery. I also called my parents, who decided to come straight up to the hospital to see me when I came around.

It wasn't long before two doctors in green surgical scrubs and clogs appeared at the door and came in to introduce themselves. As soon as the formalities were out of the way, I was shocked to hear that they didn't want to operate on me after all. They reiterated that due to the size of the infection inside my appendix there may be complications, which could result in a prolonged stay in hospital fighting infection. They also told me that their planned keyhole surgery may have to be abandoned for an open-cut procedure if they ran into any difficulties. I got the distinct impression that they were not keen at all.

I asked what the alternative would be and they suggested more antibiotics and a further consultation in a month. I was struggling to process the conversation quickly enough to really grasp what they were saying and I was just about to agree, albeit reluctantly, to go home with some more painkillers when I was thrown a lifeline: 'But of course, it's entirely up to you. If you want to proceed today we are happy to go ahead, as long as you understand the risks.'

I asked when they thought the operation would go ahead if we cancelled.

'As long as the infection is clear we can schedule it in for the next six to eight weeks.'

I took a moment to think about it. I was lying on a hospital bed in a gown and pants and those bloody stupid looking compression socks with two surgeons staring at me who were prepared to operate today, or I could face an open-ended wait for another opportunity to lie in the same position in front of the same doctors. I decided to take a calculated risk and get on with it.

The decision was made, so I signed the disclaimer and was told that I would be brought down to theatre within the hour. When they left, I thought about the decision I'd made and was pleased I'd stayed strong and asked for the operation. It would have been so much easier to agree with their obviously preferred option and get dressed and go home. Whatever happened that afternoon would be the end of it and I would just have to deal with any complications if they occurred.

I'd had a general anaesthetic when I donated bone marrow a few years ago and also when I had my tonsils removed in my 20s, so I knew what to expect as I was wheeled down to the theatre by the porter. I know that any operation carries risk but I wasn't feeling particularly worried, I resolved to just enjoy the ride and let the doctors do the worrying.

Things happen alarmingly fast when you arrive in theatre. You go crashing through the swinging saloon doors into a kind of holding area where the theatre nurses and the anaesthetist always greet you with beaming smiles. They try to be as jolly as possible to keep you calm, as they check the paperwork to make sure you are who you are supposed to be. I didn't want to be mixed up with the bloke in the next bay who, knowing my luck, was having his testicles removed. They then lay you back on the trolley ready to go through another set of slam doors on the opposite side of the room. That's the mystery room, you never get to see inside there as you are always long gone before you get there, well hopefully anyway. The horror stories about people being paralysed but awake through their surgeries did cross my mind at that point.

Do I need to take my pants off? 'No, you can leave them on.'

A cannula was expertly inserted within a minute of being in the room, and within another minute I was being asked to just 'lie back and relax' as the anaesthetist began pumping in the milky anaesthetic. The sensation can only be cheerfully described as what it must feel like to be dying. The world closes in very quickly from the sides, like a heavy blanket being thrown over your head. Within seconds a metallic taste had spread through my mouth and I managed to say out loud, 'Oh, I can taste ...'

The next thing I remembered was waking up with a start in the recovery area with a nurse calling my name. I stared around blinking and feeling disorientated. I was having a really vivid psychedelic dream which I instantly managed to forget the moment I woke up. My mouth was bone dry and my tongue was stuck inside my cheek as I tried to talk. I took a sip of water and lay back again on the bed. Naturally the first thing you ask is 'how did it go?'

'Very well, by all accounts, it was a difficult operation and took longer than expected but they are very happy with the outcome. The consultant will visit you and discuss the details when you are back on the ward.'

I peered under the sheet and pulled up my gown. I could see three dressings with little blood dots in the middle of them stuck to my brown iodine-stained abdomen, so it was by keyhole after all then.

I was allowed to come around gently and was then wheeled back up to my room in the same bed and allowed to sleep for a bit. I was relieved that I had gone through with it. I imagined myself taking the other course of action and being back at home taking an endless supply of horse-sized antibiotics whilst my appendix slowly poisoned me.

My surgeon appeared later that evening and explained that the operation went very well. It was more complicated than usual as the infection was widespread and my body had created a fatty layer over my entire appendix to seal in the infection. Due to this, the fatty layer was stuck down along the length of my bowel and was even attached to my liver, meaning a small piece of liver had to be removed with it.

I was told that I would be monitored in hospital for a couple of days until I had passed a stool and I needed to take it easy until my wounds had healed, due to the risk of a hernia. I would be given regular painkillers and antibiotics to ensure that any residual infection cleared up.

I was pleased that my appendix was gone at last and I could recover and get back to work and, more importantly, back to some sort of exercise. All this time off had really dented any hopes I had of doing any type of event that summer, or for that matter any exercise at all, let alone to start to train for an Ironman.

That evening the nurse was reviewing my file and I glimpsed some photos taken during my operation. I asked if I could take a look. It was fascinating to see just what the fuss had been about. You could clearly see my appendix stuck to my bowel and where it had been burnt away to remove it. I had to have a copy of those, so I asked for a print but the nurse said it wasn't allowed. I was gutted. 'How about I just photograph those images with my phone?' She reluctantly agreed and I was chuffed to be able to preserve the evidence; neither of us knew at that time what we were really looking at in those photos.

Diagnosis Day

IT WASN'T long before I was back walking the same corridors again for my routine four-week post-treatment check-up. I'd been given another course of strong antibiotics which seemed to have done the trick and my keyhole surgery scars had healed well. I'd had no recurrence of the bowel pains and was feeling bright and fit as I got up that sunny morning of 6 August 2014 (some dates just stick).

It was a lovely day and as parking was such a nightmare around the hospital, I thought I'd give my motorcycle a spin as it had been languishing sadly in the garage throughout the whole of my treatment period. I fancied a decent ride, so I went the long way to the hospital and clocked a few miles with the sun and wind in my face.

I felt relaxed, happy and actually pretty refreshed; on reflection it felt like I'd just had three weeks' extra summer holiday from work, albeit sore ones.

I was sure that the appointment would be a quick in-and-out to have a look at my scars and congratulate me on a quick and successful recovery. I was the first in after lunch, so hopefully there would be no delays. I arrived at the hospital in plenty of time, parked up and made my way to the waiting room. My god, it was hot and busy in there. I checked in with the receptionist and peeling off my sweaty biking gear, grabbed a water and a dog-eared copy of *Hello* from 2012 and settled in for a wait. There was a handwritten notice scrawled on the whiteboard which stated, unsurprisingly, that there was approximately an hour delay in the schedule.

I heard my name called and the duty nurse pointed me towards one of the consulting rooms, so I grabbed my helmet and walked in. I was surprised to be greeted by the same consultant who had tried to convince me to cancel my operation and go home the month before. I smiled to myself as I shook his hand, thinking that I had got one over on him by insisting that the operation went ahead and was a success after all.

As he shook my hand he looked down at my other which was clutching my motorcycle helmet. I was expecting a cheerful hello but the first thing he said was, 'Oh… you've come on a motorcycle. Is anyone with you?' I don't know if my job as a police officer has anything to do with it but I do have a nose for trouble and this stank of it from the moment I walked into that room.

The consultant introduced me to a young doctor who was assisting him for the day and, looking decidedly uncomfortable, she smiled awkwardly as we exchanged greetings with a particularly limp handshake. We sat down and looking at them I knew something bad was coming and the wait for it was already feeling like a long one.

'So Mr Smith, how have you been feeling? I have some news to give you as we have recently received your histology results.'

'I'm ok, thank you.' … waiting …

'So how are your surgery wounds healing?' he asked.

'Very well, thank you. Do you need to have a look?'

'Yes ok then, we should do that first I suppose.'

I jumped up on to the couch and pulled up my t-shirt as he had the quickest feel around ever and said that everything looked good. 'Come and sit back at the desk please.' He was definitely distracted and this just sealed the deal for me, something serious was coming and he just needed to get on with it.

'I'm afraid I have some bad news for you. Following your appendectomy, we sent off the tissue and the results have been returned to us. Your appendix contained cancer cells.'

I raised an eyebrow quizzically and nodded in their direction, 'Ok … so what does that mean?' Unfortunately for me he didn't seem to know any more than that. He asked if I was alright and how I felt about it. To be honest at that point I was still just taking it in and didn't really have anything to add, so we just stared at each other for a bit.

He broke the silence with, 'Do you have any questions?'

'How long have I got?' I asked, trying my best to employ some wit accompanied by a shaky smile in an attempt to break the awkwardness. They didn't laugh.

'I can't answer that I'm afraid, but I believe you have some time to consider treatment options. I have made an appointment with the bowel consultant and an oncologist to discuss it further.'

I took down the dates which were in a fortnight's time back at the hospital. At least they didn't appear to think I was going to be dead before then.

'So, will I be needing chemotherapy then?' I asked.

'Maybe.'

'So what type of cancer is it?'

'I can't say at this time.'

'Will it kill me?'

'Again, further tests and a treatment plan will have to be agreed.'

The non-committal replies were giving me no clues. It was abundantly clear that I wasn't going to be getting any decent answers out of the two cardboard cut-outs propped up opposite me, so I would just have to be content with the news that I had cancer while I waited for the next fortnight to see a doctor who may know a bit more.

The consultation then wrapped up pretty quickly.

'Anyone we can call for you? Will you be alright getting home?'

'I'll be fine, thank you.' There were more limp handshakes all round and I thanked them both and left. What was that all about?

'Thanks for telling me I've got cancer.'

'No problem Mr Smith, my pleasure, take care.'

Blimey, us Brits are far too polite sometimes. I tumbled back into the heat of the reception area and it instantly felt like everyone was staring at me.

'Poor lad,' 'so young,' 'he's not going to ride that motorcycle home is he?'

I returned to the reception desk to collect a copy of the letter for my next consultation. The receptionist flashed me a caring smile, she definitely knew. I took it, thanked her and strode out of the hospital back into the sunshine.

I found a bench outside and took a few minutes in the sun to digest what I'd just been told. Maria had been away with work for a couple of nights and was coming back on the train that evening – once again I had managed to convince her that she didn't need to be there. I would have to think of a way of telling her. Oh fuck, and my parents, that wasn't going to be easy.

I felt weirdly detached, as if I was in a dream. I imagined that I should be crying my eyes out and terrified, but I was surprisingly calm. I couldn't work out why I wasn't more emotional. It felt like a story that was happening to somebody else. Maybe it was the lack of information – I couldn't be frightened of something I knew nothing about – but what I did know was that there were going to be some significant changes in my life and perhaps even in my life expectancy. I felt like I was standing on the edge in a blindfold – was I about to step off the kerb or a cliff? Without knowing which, how could I be scared?

I was bursting to tell someone, but who do you call in times like these? I've only got one person who gets all the breaking news and juicy gossip from me and that's my best friend of 20-odd years Luigi, so I rang him. 'Mate. Can you talk for a minute?' I knew he was at work so not the ideal time to drop the 'C bomb' but hey, he's my best mate and he would just have to suck it up.

I told him what went down and he was clearly shocked but was very cool. I ran past him a plan about how I would tell Maria and we agreed to catch up properly the next day. In all honesty there wasn't that much to say as I didn't have any details to give him.

As I sat there outside the hospital, I watched some clearly very ill people walking in and out and wondered how long it would be until I was one of them. I was still surprised how calm I was. I had a moment when the bottom lip wobbled and a couple of tears squeezed out, but that was thinking about Maria's reaction and not in self-pity. I've always considered myself to have a very even temperament, I've never been one for big emotional swings or outbursts of anger or upset. Maria, with her hot-blooded Eastern European temperament, would get annoyed with me because I never rose to her when she was spoiling for a fight – the best stab at being emotional I could muster was puffing out my cheeks and sighing.

I had about four hours before she got off the train, so I jumped back on the motorbike and blasted out for another long run home via the countryside. I sent her a text message when I got back and said I would meet her at the train station.

The sun was still shining, so I changed into shorts and a t-shirt and walked into town. As I walked I started perfecting my plan of how to tell my wife that I had cancer without alarming her and without being able to give her any more information than just that – it wasn't going to be an easy task.

My plan was to meet her at the station and suggest a walk and something to eat in town as it was such a nice evening. I'd take her to the park, sit her down on the grass and just come out with it and take it from there. Good plan, I thought.

I was early so I sat in a pub garden in the sun and had a couple of pints while I watched the world go by; I'm not one for Dutch courage but I thought I'd treat myself in the circumstances. I sat and listened to some heavy metal on the iPod and shed another couple of tears behind my sunglasses. I could sense that the bloke sat at the next table was itching to ask me if I was alright, so I downed my pint and left, walking the long way to the train station.

I glimpsed her in the rush-hour crowd coming through the exit barrier long before she saw me and walked towards her. She spotted me and flashed me a broad smile. We hugged and before I could say anything she said, 'How are you doing? How did you get on at the hospital?' Bugger.

'I'm alright, yes all good,' I choked. 'Fancy going for a walk as it's such a nice evening?' She agreed and with a sigh of relief my plan was initiated. We walked through town to the park and she must have asked me a dozen times if I was alright. I think she knew I was acting a bit weird and she probably guessed that I'd be surprising her with something at some point, no shit.

We found a spot on the grass, sat down and I just came out with it. She stared at me, reached out and held my hand and cried. I tried to play it down. I felt healthy, we didn't know the details, there was no rush to see the consultant but it really wasn't working. We both knew that a page had turned and the future was, for now at the very least, uncertain.

That's when the smart move would have been to go home, but I was pushing on with the plan and wanted the evening to be as normal as possible so I continued to stage two and suggested we go to a nearby restaurant. She agreed and we ate a pretty tasteless meal, sat in near silence. The reality was settling in and poor Maria was choking back tears whilst trying not to make a fuss in a busy eatery. A lot of eyes were on us and they must have wondered what the hell was going on. I have since been quite rightly blamed for ruining the ambience at one of her favourite restaurants.

Afterwards we walked home in the warmth of the evening and reflected on what the future could bring. I agreed to tell my family in person at the weekend and called my parents to say we were coming down for a visit.

We went to bed and cuddled, nothing further was said but I could feel the wet tickle of a tear on my collarbone as I lay holding her in the dark. I felt overwhelmingly sorry for her but surprisingly I still felt no self-pity. It was at that moment lying in the dark that I made a contract with myself. I wasn't dying yet, I was fit and active and in no pain. I would not allow myself to get negative and I would do everything I could to be ready for any treatment I needed. I was 43 and I'd had a good life. I wasn't a child dying of some disease, I wasn't an 18-year-old soldier dying in a war and I hadn't been snatched away after being run over by a bus. I had a lot to be grateful for and a lot of living still to do.

In the time-honoured fashion for all cancer victims, I was going to fight it. Fuck you, cancer.

I lay and listened to Maria's breathing get heavier as she fell asleep then allowed myself to drift off. I was exhausted and I slept like a log.

Seeing your Parents Can Be a Real Pain

BEING DIAGNOSED with cancer makes you think back on all the tell-tale signs that may have told you that there was something more going on than just a bit of wind.

My big 'oh shit, that's what that must have been' moment was reflecting back to a visit to my parents in the summer of 2013. It was a hot weekend and they live near the coast, so we had packed up the car for some time at the beach and for being fed and watered by my mum.

We arrived on the Friday evening and I was already starting to feel a bit bloated and uncomfortable after dinner. It was hot and I spent the evening lying awkwardly on the sofa trying to squeeze out a fart which just wasn't coming. I went to bed still feeling bloated but thought that a good shit the next morning would sort me out.

My apologies to anyone who may be put off by the talk of my bowel movements, but when the subject matter of this book is going to be bowel cancer, you need to trust me when I say it's going to get a lot worse from here on in.

The next morning I wasn't feeling much better but we went to the beach anyway and had a good day out, but the whole time I was feeling hot and thirsty and a cramping pain down my right side was starting to develop. I was still feeling bloated but wasn't so uncomfortable that I needed to make a fuss or say anything to my wife.

The dull ache stayed in the background with the bloating, but I did feel better after I had let out a very long, low fart as I hung back from Maria on the walk back to the car. Maybe I was just dehydrated and some water would do the trick.

Mum always does a killer roast (probably a poor choice of words) and as a greedy bugger I wasn't going to be missing out on a leg of lamb because of a bit of stomach ache. I have a good appetite and as usual I managed seconds of everything. I knew as soon as I finished that I had made a mistake by having such a big dinner.

The pain in my right side intensified to a stabbing, pulsing cramp within about 30 minutes of finishing. I laid out on the sofa and just couldn't get comfortable, so I said to Maria that we should probably go home as I wasn't feeling well. I had a proper sweat going on by this point and Mum felt bad because she thought she'd poisoned me.

Maria drove us back as I wasn't feeling up to it. Her driving has been known to make me feel unwell at the best of times but as we sat in the car in the heat of what felt like an endless Sunday traffic jam, I knew that there was something more serious happening to me. I was squirming around in the car seat as severe stabbing pains shot around inside me. They were all emanating from my lower right-hand side and I immediately suspected appendicitis.

As I've said, it takes a lot for any man to take himself to the doctor's but I was well and truly considering it by the time we were an hour into the journey. I turned to Maria and said that she should probably take me straight to the hospital when we got back. She was already worried about me and that alarming revelation certainly upped the ante somewhat. Of all the things to come out of my mouth, that certainly isn't the first she would have thought of. We drove straight to accident and emergency and it was five o'clock on the dot as we parked up, so hopefully it wasn't going to be too busy.

We staggered through the doors with me huffing and puffing and hanging off Maria's arm and as soon as we got inside we were hit by the waft of hot smelly bodies and a stench of general misery. Looking around, every seat was taken in the waiting area by bored, glassy-eyed people, half of whom looked like they probably shouldn't have even been there.

We shuffled up to the desk to check in only to be told that the wait was up to six hours if it wasn't urgent. As I was still standing/talking/breathing a little bit of tummy ache wasn't going to get me to the front of the queue. The receptionist had a cunning plan, though; the on-call doctors' surgery was open in maternity next door and I could check in there as the wait was only going to be two or three hours.

The atmosphere of despair was slightly less palpable in the doctors' waiting area but the temperature was right up into sauna-like proportions. The clientele here were decidedly more downmarket as well. The sweet smell of alcohol, stale cigarettes and body odour from an afternoon of barbecuing formed the overwhelming top note to the stifling ambience, but at least we could get a seat in there.

After three hours of listening to sewer-mouthed people moaning about the state of the National Health Service, whilst marching back and forth to the reception to demand a reason why their snotty little darlings weren't being seen quickly enough, I was just about ready to go home. I was still feeling decidedly uncomfortable but the painful stabbing pains I was having earlier had begun to subside. There's something about being at the doctor's that instantly makes you feel as if you are getting better and wasting everyone's time.

Just as I was about to lose my cool with my fellow patients and say something I might regret, I was called forward. The doctor was pleasant enough but I could tell he was underwhelmed as I presented myself. He had a good feel and asked if I'd been breaking wind and had passed a stool. I had, of course, done both and as I wasn't writhing in agony by that stage even I had the distinct feeling that I was making a fuss.

'Well that's all good,' said the doctor. 'You could have a bit of a blockage or a twisted bowel. We can admit you tonight for observations or if you are feeling up to it you can go home and come back in if it gets any worse. Take these pills which should help get you going again.'

The prospect of a night in hospital wasn't particularly appealing so I took the pills along with my chances and went home. We were knackered as it was well after midnight when we got in, so we went straight to bed. I woke up and of course felt much better. 'That's a relief, thank god that's all over with,' I said to Maria, and with that I took myself back off to work.

Making Sense of the Big C

YOU GET told you've got cancer and then you have to wait a fortnight before you get to hear any details whatsoever about it – what sort of a sick joke is that? What the hell do you do to keep yourself sane in the meantime? A bit of internet research was in order.

Cancer has a certain image, don't you think? I'd say that its fearsome reputation has been well-earned by being the number-one dealer of slow lingering deaths with endless people withering away in a hospice somewhere – a horrifying prospect.

There is another side to cancer though, a hopeful future brought on by constant advances in treatments and clinical trials.

The news is full of stories about people who have made miraculous recoveries from a helpless terminal diagnosis, but the news is also full of stories of people dying young from cancer. Children, teenagers, young adults and celebrities all snatched away from their promising lives before their time, some long before me, that was for sure.

You quickly realise that cancer is everywhere. It's the human disease, in all its glorious multicoloured forms, striking young and old alike; it plucks people away left, right and centre. Why don't we know more about this? And why aren't we talking about this more?

It's like when you buy a new car, before you bought it you hardly saw one on the road and when you get yours, everyone has got one. I saw cancer every time I opened a newspaper and every time I turned on the television, I still do.

So, if this is cancer and I have got cancer how the fuck am I supposed to process it when I don't have a single fact about what is wrong with me other than I've got cancer, and it was on my appendix? My appendix has been taken out though, right? Doesn't this mean that it's all gone already?

Let's start with some Googling then, shall we.

What is appendix cancer?

Appendix cancer is rare, occurring in about 1,000 people in the United States each year. In those cases, abnormal cells grow wildly in your appendix (a small pouch connected to your colon with no known purpose) and form a tumour. Tumours can be either benign (non-cancerous) or malignant (cancerous).

Well that was enlightening, let's try something else.

What are the survival rates for appendix cancer?

If the tumour is no larger than three centimetres, with or without spreading to other parts of the body, the five-year survival rate is 78 per cent. If the cancer has spread to other parts of the body, the five-year survival rate is 32 per cent. Due to the rare nature of appendix cancer, specific statistics are not available.

Fuck that, 32 per cent for only five years. I'll just wait for the doctor to tell me what's what. I knew that the internet was not going to help much but you can't help but look. We all know that if you type 'sore throat' into a search engine you get told to see your doctor because you might be dying.

But 32 per cent for five years though, there it is again. It kept popping up in my head. Once you've seen a statistic like that you just can't un-see it.

What else does it say? If the tumour is bigger than three centimetres. Tick. What about if it has spread to other parts of the body? I had that bloody drain put in, that must have caused some damage to the sack around my appendix and I had been told it had burst anyway. It was touching my liver, that constitutes spreading surely? The cancer might have come out of my appendix and spread from there – 32 per cent – I certainly wasn't prepared to dig out my old Dungeons and Dragons dice and roll out those odds just yet.

Suddenly you find yourself carving your life into five-year slices, five years. Fuck off, that's no time at all. What if half of that is lived in agony from inoperable tumours.

Can another five years really be all I've got? Who knows? It was only the other day in work we were talking about how long it is till we can retire and moaning about it being a long way away. I'll take that long wait right now, thank you. It's very easy to mark time in life and wish it away. If I do get told I've got five years, what the hell am I going to do with them?

It felt like the breath of the Grim Reaper on my neck and it gave me goosebumps. He's not ready to take me just yet, as he's just finishing up scything down some other poor sod, but he wants me to know he's coming. In that moment you have to rewire your brain and educate yourself very quickly to make sense of what life really is and what it really means to you to be alive.

The conclusion I came to is that cancer is a bit of a dirty secret that other people get and we don't really want to talk about it. Why would we spend emotional energy thinking about this disease and confronting the possibility that we could all get it? Death is that old elephant in the room and no one likes to think about that, but suddenly it's the only thing I can think about.

The clichés are all lined up ready for us: life's too short, live the dream, seize the day. The problem is we don't. We should do all these things every day, not just as we have some epiphany when it's too late.

In those first few days I heard people saying things like 'Why you, it's so unfair,' but is it really? What's unfair about it? It's just life dealing its hand, surely. If not me then who? And why not me? What makes me more deserving than some toddler fighting for their life somewhere?

I needed to start dealing with my thoughts by being positive, so I made a start. I may have cancer but I'm not sick yet. Over time that line became my mantra. I wasn't dying at that very moment and I wouldn't be for a while yet, so that surely gave me a fighting chance.

I was in better shape now that the appendicitis was dealt with than I had been in a good few years. I also had choices – I could sit back in some self-induced pity party or I could start doing something to prepare for whatever it was that was coming my way. Fitness was already starting to play a part in my life before this news and it would be fitness that would give me purpose and drive, right up until a doctor told me otherwise.

If I needed chemotherapy or another operation I would need to be in the best physical shape of my life. Never mind doing an Ironman, this was the real event and one I knew I would have to face head-on over the next few weeks if I was going to give myself the best chance I could.

I was fighting on two fronts from the moment I was given the diagnosis. I was fighting the cancer both mentally and physically and I needed a strategy to cope with both equally. I had already decided that I couldn't allow myself to slip into self-pity and was working out in my head what positive steps I could take to prevent it. Any thoughts of self-pity I did harbour irritated me immensely and made me angry with myself for entertaining them. If anyone else expressed a similar sentiment on behalf of me, or themselves, I absolutely hated it. I would tell people that I didn't feel bitter about it so no one else should either.

The problem with that type of mindset was that it didn't allow people around me to express themselves for fear of upsetting me and I found that people often held in their own feelings about what was happening for my sake. Maria had to be particularly strong for me around this time. In hindsight I wouldn't have been so zealous about it all, but at the end of the day it was me with the cancer, not them, and it was me who had to find a path through it, so I made it damn clear that there would be no pity in any shape or form around me.

Physically, I was aware of the head start I had over some people in a similar position to me. I may have been carrying a few extra pounds, but I was reasonably fit and had a flying start at this. If I didn't take advantage of my position on the starting grid then who could I blame if I didn't make it because of the shape I was in? This was a very cold reality for me. I've said before I was a bit of a lazy bastard at heart and I had to confront that attitude head on. If this wasn't the wake-up call I needed then what the hell was going to be?

I needed to be very clear from the start. This was going to be a fight for my life, THE fight for my life. When it's cold and wet outside are you really going to roll over, turn off the alarm and have a lie-in? It's a bloody long lie-in when you're dead, that's for sure.

Keeping positive is much more about deeds than thoughts, so it was time to have another look at that triathlon training plan and make a fresh start from the beginning. No one had told me I was going to die just yet so I tried not to worry about it until they did.

Keep Calm and Swim

I'D DONE all my thinking and I knew that being the fittest I could be for any treatment ahead was absolutely the best thing I could do for myself. It would keep me sane by giving me something to focus on and an achievement to aim for, but I really needed to set some benchmarks. I needed a goal otherwise, being my own worst enemy, I wasn't at the point where I could fully trust myself to just go out and do some exercise without a plan to stick to.

I have always been very much a to-do list kind of person. I find it hard to concentrate and focus on a task if I don't have it laid out in front of me in bite-size pieces to tick off.

At work I have the habit of writing a to-do list virtually every day. I can put in that list all the shitty jobs which I would normally put to the back of the pile and it helps me to get on with them when they are staring me in the face every day until they are done. I always feel a sense of achievement ticking off or striking through the things on my lists.

I needed a focussed programme and the one Tom and I had been flirting with in work all year seemed the perfect place to start.

Don Fink in his book *Be Iron Fit* breaks the training for an Ironman into three distinct ten-week phases. The first of these is the base phase and is designed to get you fit enough to train six days a week without injury. The programme is progressive and works within heart rate zones, ensuring that whilst you are completing such an arduous task as an Ironman, you will always be operating in a comfortable zone without going into the red if possible. The theory being that if you are always working at a sustainable level and you continue to fuel yourself, you can go on indefinitely.

Being a triathlon plan, it obviously focusses on the three disciplines of swimming, cycling and running. Now I am no accomplished athlete, but in two of these disciplines I could safely say I had some limited experience. I'd run a few ten kilometre events, two half-marathons and even cycled a few 65-mile sportives, and completed some long solo bike rides. So I knew what it meant to follow a progressive training programme in these sports. I owned a half-decent, carbon-fibre-framed road bike and some properly fitting trainers, so I was ready to roll in these disciplines.

Swimming, on the other hand, was going to be a bit of a problem.

This is definitely the time to explain my relationship with swimming: I don't really swim. In fact, I can safely say that I don't like swimming. No, that's not strong enough, I hate swimming. If I'm completely honest, I've always been a bit scared of swimming. There you go I've said it, that's the truth of it and the reason I've been avoiding swimming since I was a kid.

I can swim but I'm the kind of 'jump in and swim across the swimming pool once on your holiday' type of swimmer. Breaststroke only and head strictly above the water, with maybe the odd star float and a quick bit of front crawl whilst holding my breath and thrashing like I'm about to drown or like I'm being attacked by a shark.

My relationship with swimming has never been a good one. I remember at first school we would take an old-fashioned double-decker bus to the local leisure centre once a week for swimming lessons. Every child for a generation in our town was taught by the same swimming teacher, Mr Bird. I can see him now, too-tight red shorts and hairy legs with a massive Leo Sayer style perm and a whistle on a lanyard which he would blow furiously when we were messing about or getting too noisy.

School swimming was graded into different certificate levels. For the beginner certificate you had to swim one width of the pool, which was ten metres, execute a front and back star float to the satisfaction of Mr Bird and then do a mushroom float. What the hell was the point of a mushroom float, bobbing in the water with your legs pulled up to your chest until you couldn't hold your breath any longer and came spluttering up to the surface? To me it only enhanced my ever-developing fear of drowning.

I remember having the test for my beginner certificate during our very first lesson. A whole class of skinny, shivering kids waited their turn to jump in at the sound of the whistle to do their width. I stood in that line confident I could move straight into the intermediate group with the rest of my friends as I had done a bit of swimming with my dad and the Cub Scouts.

My turn came and I jumped in and started to swim. I got halfway across and was already starting to get tired. Come on Paul you can do this, don't panic. I started to thrash around just wanting it to be done, not far to go now. I could hear a whistle frantically blowing and looked over to see Mr Bird pointing at me from the side of the pool. I stopped and stood up to my waist in the shallow end. 'NO BACKSTROKE! YOU HAVE TO DO IT ON YOUR FRONT,' he was shouting. I had to wade all the way back and start again. I hate you.

I was crestfallen and exhausted. There was no way I could manage that, and I didn't. The plucky six-year-old me did give it a go, though, and nearly drowned in the process. I watched as all my friends and 95 per cent of the class easily progressed to the intermediate group as I was left floundering in the beginners with, quite frankly, the bottom five per cent of kids in all departments. You know the sort, the ones you didn't invite to your birthday party, and now I was one of them, and I wasn't happy about it.

I don't think that the scars inflicted on my subconscious on that traumatic day ever healed and I never felt the love for the water from that day forth. It took the rest of that school term for me to join the others in the intermediates, just as they all left for the advanced group in the deep pool. The 1970s was a pretty uncompromising decade for education – if you didn't make the grade you would be easily forgotten about in the remedial groups. Mr Bird was always blowing his whistle up the other end of the pool where the smarter, more capable kids were doing cool things like diving off the springboard. Me and my new best friends were left to thrash around doing our own thing in the shallows while one of our teachers, who should have been monitoring us, took a nap on the bench.

Everyone, when asked about school swimming lessons, will talk fondly of retrieving plastic bricks from the bottom of the pool in their pyjamas. The sad truth is I never got to do any of that because it was as good as I could manage to swim out of my depth for ten seconds before I had a panic attack. I would stick to the side of the pool with all the plasters, pubes and chewing gum as if my life depended on it. I was such a terrible swimmer I reckon I would have drowned in the medicated foot bath in front of the changing rooms if I were wearing my pyjamas.

So that was that, my swimming fate was sealed. I could swim to save my life but not a lot more, and I was destined to swim breaststroke like an old lady for the rest of my days. I may as well have been done with it and bought one of those plastic swim caps with the flowers on it.

Nothing like piling pressure on myself, then. If I was serious about doing a triathlon I would have to learn to swim.

I didn't have any proper swimming kit though, and if I was going to do this properly I would need some good-quality swimming equipment. My desire for new sports kit was reignited and that went some way to placating my fear of getting in the water and actually doing it. Tom had loaned me his copy of *Swim Smooth*, another fitness bible to digest and follow. So into the internet I delved and ordered some decent swimming trunks, goggles, swim fins for leg drills and a pull buoy for arm exercises. No excuses now then, all the gear and all that.

My first training session after my diagnosis was to be a swim, a deliberate ploy to force myself to get on with it.

So on the Wednesday evening I went with Maria to the local 20m pool and literally took the plunge. I was nervous on the drive up but didn't want to say anything to my wife, who is a ridiculously smooth swimmer. As we walked through the doors, that familiar warm swimming pool smell of chlorine and musty changing rooms washed over me. I felt a bit queasy and I really wasn't looking forward to it one bit.

In the changing rooms I was all fingers and thumbs as I fumbled around getting changed and I could feel my heart pounding in my chest. Come on Smith, this is ridiculous, get a grip of yourself. I walked out and stepped under a cruelly cold shower before walking across to sit on the edge of the pool. It was busy. There were lots of pensioners in the pool that evening for some reason and I had to scour around for a suitable spot for me to swim in. Some swimmers were evidently too slow and they needed to be avoided and others seemed to be swimming very smoothly in their lanes and I would surely be just getting in their way.

I knew I was already overthinking it and just had to get in and start swimming. I pulled my goggles down and slid into the water. I started with a length of breaststroke, instantly reverting to type with the pensioners around me. By the time I'd got back to where I started after negotiating two lengths, I was breathing quite heavily and felt pretty knackered. I rested for a minute and then did the same again. This time I could already feel the muscles across my chest and shoulders pulling.

I gave it another couple of minutes and stretched out in the water while I worked out in my head how I was going to tackle my first lengths of front crawl. I had read some of *Swim Smooth* and knew that technique was everything, including breathing to both sides. I knew in my head what I thought a decent stroke looked like, so I just needed to stop messing about and try it.

Head down in the water, I pushed off from the side and took my first gliding stroke. I was swimming and it felt alright. I could see the end of the length in front of me and as I neared it I could feel the old panic starting to rise. I was badly struggling for breath and the six-year-old in me began thrashing for the safety of the end of the pool. I made it and was breathing really hard. I'd swam the whole length without taking a single breath and it was hard work.

I looked across and Maria was gliding through the fast lane. I told myself again to get a grip, the more I did this the easier it would become. I swam back in the same breathless manner and halfway across as I rolled to the side to take a breath I gulped in a lungful of water. I spluttered and coughed under the water and my foot instantly went down. I stood up and was massively disappointed in myself. Is that as good as it gets for me, I thought? I coughed the water out of my lungs and nose and swam for the end. I grabbed the side of the pool and floated for a bit, getting my breath and composure back.

I did a grand total of 16 lengths of the 20m pool that first evening, and each one was as hideous as the last. I was both mentally and physically exhausted by the time we left.

What the hell was I doing thinking about triathlons when my swimming was this bad? I had to remind myself that this was all part of the challenge and it wasn't going to come easily. I had to embrace the pool and start to enjoy it if I was going to win this battle.

To hit those swimming demons head on, I went back the next day, but on my own this time. The pool was a lot quieter and already felt a little more familiar. I swam another 14 lengths in a similarly poor fashion as the day before but I did have my pull buoy with me this time and, tucking it firmly between my legs, it at least allowed me to swim a few consecutive lengths whilst actually breathing.

I left the pool that evening feeling a little more optimistic. I knew that I had a huge amount of work to do but I could see that, with some perseverance, swimming more than one length at a time was probably doable and that was a good start in my book.

What struck me the most as I drove home that evening was the fact that I had been concentrating so hard whilst in the water, I didn't think about the cancer once and that alone had to be worth going back for.

Kicking off a Ten-Week Block

NO MORE messing around, it was time to knuckle down and get this ten-week training plan off the ground and in the meantime, if I was very lucky, find out if I was likely to live to see the end of that ten weeks. It was going to be a busy few weeks and ones which would probably shape the rest of my long, or short, life.

I was still in good spirits despite the obvious worry about what might happen to me festering away in the back of my mind. I was a little surprised that these feelings weren't clamouring to overwhelm me, but in reality they weren't even coming close. I've said before that I'm generally quite calm in a crisis, but this was new and uncharted territory and I needed to process why I was feeling like I was.

I found it strange that I wasn't panicking. I was still sleeping really well and still enjoying all the talk of an Ironman at work and thinking about the challenge of the training programme I was embarking on. I'd ask myself if I was in some sort of denial but the more I thought about it the less likely that seemed to be. My old mantra of 'no one has told you you're dying yet' was helping a lot, and, even though the reality was that no one had told me anything yet, I was determined to deal with each challenge as it occurred and not before.

As a treat to ourselves, Maria and I took the opportunity in the two weekends after the diagnosis to go away somewhere nice to try to relax and unwind. We spent fantastic weekends in Oxford and Bath and this helped to both distract us and give us some quality time to talk openly about it all in a different environment over a few cocktails and a nice meal. The result was well worth the expense, as we both came back from those weekends feeling refreshed and pampered with a renewed sense of togetherness and focus.

I was now swimming two or three times a week, and although I was hating every bloody minute of it I could feel the progress, and despite my reticence there was no way I was going to be a triathlete, let alone an Ironman, if I didn't get to grips with it. My training sessions were mostly lonely thrashings amongst the old-aged pensioners at the local pool, but my swim training was about to ratchet itself up several notches on the fear factor.

Open-water swimming, bloody hell what was I thinking? It was another essential ingredient in the skill set of a triathlete. I had seen an advert for an offer on wetsuits in a triathlon magazine a couple of weeks before and pulled the trigger and went for it. I bought one for both my wife and myself, along with some decent goggles and a swim cap. My love of kit had once again been indulged and we even had a swimming lake very close to us where apparently the first-ever UK triathlon took place back in the early 1980s, so we were all set to go.

The wetsuits were duly delivered and I was keen to get into mine. When you research about swimming wetsuits they are very different beasts to the bullet-proof wetsuits I was used to surfing in. The surface of the suit is smooth to aid your glide through the water. They have thicker neoprene in the legs for buoyancy (I liked the sound of that) but they were paper thin on the surface and prone to tearing, and they were also bloody hard to get into.

Ten minutes of tugging, pulling and hopping around on one leg and I'd got it halfway up my chest. Trying to get my arms in was like getting into a straitjacket, but eventually I got it on with an elastic twang. I was standing in the middle of the lounge sweating and wheezing – I could barely stand up straight in the thing, it was so tight over my shoulders and chest. I shuffled over to look at myself in the mirror. What confronted me was, quite frankly, disgusting. Despite being the tightest thing you could possibly compress your body into, it did nothing to hide the curves. I stood hunched forward, looking like some sort of red-faced gimp who'd forgotten his mask and stared at the pretty pronounced pot belly that was poking out at me. Surely I wasn't that fat? I looked like a black pudding. Thank fuck I would be spending most of my time up to my neck in the water as this thing was not flattering in the least.

Now that was a point, the water. How the hell was I going to swim in this thing when I couldn't even stand up straight in it? I remembered the mushroom float from my childhood and suddenly realised a use for it but I wasn't going to swim far with the body shape of a cooked prawn.

With some assistance from Maria, who had, without fuss, quietly managed to slip into hers, we managed to yank it up high enough for me to straighten my back and move my arms around. The resulting camel toe and wedgie was taking my breath away, but I took comfort that I had read somewhere that it would apparently loosen up a bit when wet.

Another thankfully shorter battle then ensued to get the thing off, during which it felt like I was trying to escape the clutches of a massive boa constrictor. Suddenly I was free from it and as I kicked it off my foot and stood dripping in sweat in just my underpants, I wondered how I was supposed to manage exercising in it when I was that exhausted just getting in and out of it.

I'd now started adding the run and cycle elements to my training, and, although they were fairly easy sessions at this stage, they were going to plan, which felt great. I had thought about some strength training, but after attempting a plank one evening in the bedroom and ending up collapsing in an agonising naked heap after just one second, I thought better of it. I'd had no appreciation of what the surgery had done to my abs until that point, and realised I would have to build it up slowly. As a side note, I still believe it was attempting a 30-day plank challenge that squeezed and burst my appendix in the first place.

After one particularly sweaty run of about three miles, I got back and my abs were killing me. I still had the remainder of my stitches dissolving and falling out from my keyhole surgery scars and I could feel a hard lump under one of the left-hand scars. I squeezed it and out popped a large glob of pus. I knew then that I was going to have to temper my training to how I was mending and how I was feeling, and I wondered how I was going to get on after the more invasive surgery or chemotherapy that was likely to be happening soon. I thought back to my favourite mantra and told myself to take one step at a time and not waste my energy worrying.

With the cycling back on track, it was time to think about a new bike. The bike I was riding was a half-decent full carbon-framed racer with a reasonable level of kit on it, but it was cheap, and in my book cheap might have been cheerful but it was certainly not the bike to be showing off around other triathletes at the lake, or one to propel me on to triathlon glory. So the search was on. It had served me well on the few sportives I'd entered in the past, but being a confirmed poser meant that if I was serious about cycling I should look the part. The 'rules' of cycling are very important to performance and general well-being. If you don't know the rules, type 'Velominati' into the internet and check them out.

As luck would have it, Tom, as usual, knew someone who knew someone who was selling a bike. It was a Cannondale SuperSix racing bike in my size and was perfect for me. Apparently the chap had bought it with a few tasty upgrades about a year before with the intention of becoming the next Bradley Wiggins, but after falling off it and being completely physically destroyed on an inappropriately long maiden ride with his friends, he had lost the love and it was now up for sale having sat forlornly in his garage for the year. He wanted half of what he paid for it, which was still about all I had to spend on a new bike anyway. It seemed too good a deal to get twice the bike for my budget and I didn't take much convincing as it was a lovely bike and had great reviews. It was perfect for triathlon and especially Ironman.

A deal was struck and within two weeks I had rushed down with Tom between jobs at work to fetch it and it was back in my garage and ready for action. I can honestly say that it has been excellent to me from day one. I still have it and still love to ride it as much as I love to just look at it, a very worthwhile treat for a man with cancer. I wasn't sure how long that excuse would wash with the missus, but while it lasted I needed to make the most of it and get spending.

The day was now looming for my first lake swim and I was excited and apprehensive in equal measure. I had read and been told about the buoyancy properties of swimming wetsuits, so I took confidence that my usual default position in the water of slowly sinking under the surface may be alleviated a little and make the experience if not more pleasurable, then at least less terrifying and a bit safer.

But then there was the deep dark water with actual living creatures lurking in the murk and clutching weeds which I imagined dragging me down to a watery fate. I wasn't sure how I would react to any of this, but it was certainly another distraction taking my mind off of the impending consultant's meeting, so that was all good in my book.

So what about that meeting then? Tuesday, 22 August 2014 at two in the afternoon. The day I would get to find out what was wrong with me. I'd waited what felt like an age for this day to arrive and I was hoping that I'd be given some clear idea of what to expect and the timescales involved. It felt a little weird walking back into the hospital when I was feeling so well again. I was apprehensive and strangely excited to at last get this journey underway.

Maria had taken the afternoon off work to come with me and it was another glorious day; the sun was warm on our backs as we walked into another impossibly hot hospital waiting room. The appointment was spot on time and we were ushered through to see the consultant. He rose from behind his desk to shake both our hands and introduce us to one of the cancer nurses who was also present for the meeting.

If you research what to ask at a cancer consultation on the internet you will be told to write down questions in advance so you don't forget what you want to ask. I had a few notes scribbled down but as I didn't know what to expect I found it hard to imagine what I might ask. My plan was to play it by ear and use the trusted police questioning technique of who, what, where, when, why and how to hopefully get me by.

The waistcoated consultant was very pleasant and explained that he was an experienced bowel surgeon who would be responsible for my overall care, but he was only one part of a multi-disciplined team who meet regularly to discuss new cases. My case had not yet gone to the multi-disciplined team but there was a meeting the following week and I would be discussed in detail there.

He told me that I had cancer of my appendix and it did not appear to have spread further from the scans he had observed. His plan was to perform a right hemi-colectomy via keyhole surgery.

'A what?' It was the removal of the right-hand side of the large intestine where the appendix is attached to the bowel. I would be referred to an oncologist following the multi-disciplinary meeting and further tests would need to be conducted to decide if a course of chemotherapy would be appropriate. He set the date of my operation for 16 September. He was also referring my case to a consultant at the Basingstoke and North Hampshire Hospital for a second opinion and had sent them a copy of my scans.

I would also be asked to return to the hospital for a colonoscopy to determine the condition of the inside of my bowels. I didn't have to ask what that one was. Great, that was something else to look forward to.

We were then ushered into another room with the nurse who handed me a pile of generic leaflets with names like 'cancer and me' and 'your operation'. She had little else to add and promised to be in touch with some further dates for blood tests and additional scans.

So that was that and in little over 20 minutes we were hot-footing our way back out of the hospital. So what had I learnt from all that then? The disappointing answer was not a lot. It still seemed that they hadn't really discussed my case properly and couldn't give me much more detail than I already knew. This was frustrating but it was explained to us in such a matter of fact way that it seemed we were being cared for appropriately and it was pointless to get angry or upset about it.

Trying to be rational, and thinking it through, it appeared to me that if the cancer was in my appendix and they had removed it then they may have already removed the cancer. The hemicolectomy was a precaution to remove the root of the appendix, as the consultant had called it. Further tests would then reveal if it had spread and guide any further treatment I may need.

So still no news about whether I was going to die young or not. It looked like I was going to have to wait a little longer for that, unless it was going to happen on Saturday morning as I sank unseen to the bottom of the lake.

That day came quickly and it was time to literally dip my toe into the world of open-water swimming. Maria had already been a couple of times and reassured me that it was 'great' and we planned to cycle down with our good friend Scott, have a swim and then go for a bike ride with a coffee and cake stop afterwards. The lake had big yellow and orange buoys in it marking out a 750m circular circuit from the jetty. I planned to swim one lap for starters, which would smash all my previous distance records by a very long way.

As we cycled through the gates I noticed just how busy it was. This was my first time in the presence of other triathletes and I was keen to observe what they got up to in their own environment. You hear a lot about the welcoming and encouraging atmosphere around triathlons for beginners, but it felt far from welcoming around the lake that morning. Cliquey groups were laughing, joking and talking loudly about races and personal bests, and a few peole were sporting Ironman tattoos. They were a stark contrast to the silent solitary types with good bodies who were taking their session very seriously indeed. Neither group gave us or each other as much as a glance as we racked our bikes and went in to purchase our swim tokens.

I was relieved to have practised getting into my wetsuit before then, because we changed on the grass in full view of everyone else, and I had visions of balancing on one foot, half in and half out of my wetsuit while hopping down the bank and going head first into the lake. As it happened, my transition from man to walrus went quite smoothly and I gave myself a moment to get my breath back before waddling down to the jetty.

Some people were diving straight off the side into the murky water but I took the more sedate route of sitting on the edge with my legs dangling and my toes in the water while I adjusted my goggles, swim cap and nose plug. After what seemed like an age of faffing, Maria and Scott were both staring at me from the water. I couldn't put it off any longer, it was time to get in.

I slipped off the side into the water, and bloody hell it was cold. I shuddered as water ran down my back into my suit. I told myself that I would spend some time acclimatising before I went off, but as I lifted my legs to tread water they shot up behind me with all the extra buoyancy. I was so surprised to be horizontal in the water that I just blasted off as if I was swimming for my life towards the first buoy. As I swam I could see shoals of fish swimming in the reeds below me and it felt great. I couldn't believe how easy it was, I was in some sort of hysterical bliss for all of about two minutes until things started to unravel.

I looked up to see where I was going, a skill not required when you stare at the black line at the bottom of a swimming pool. I missed a breath and swallowed a massive gulp of murky water. I began spluttering and I attempted to continue swimming whilst trying to clear my throat and get some rhythm back, but it just wasn't working. The fear was beginning to rise and I could feel its icy tentacles all around me. The water beneath me had gone from a sunlit pool full of fish, to a black abyss full of weeds which were now reaching up to drag me down.

I was gasping for breath, the cold had aggravated my asthma and my chest felt like it was being squeezed in a vice. I found myself splashing around trying to right myself and keep my head above the water. I was bobbing like a cork as I wasn't used to the sensations my wetsuit was causing and I was finding it hard to even get my legs back under me to just tread water. The consequence of all this thrashing was that I just kept dunking my head under the water.

I stopped completely for a moment to get myself together and just floated. I knew there was a reason for practising that face-down star float when I was a kid. As I relaxed I found I could tread water very easily and it helped me relax even more. I soon realised that I wasn't ever going to drown wearing a wetsuit. I had an asthma inhaler up my sleeve as I knew it was going to be likely that I'd need it, so I took a couple of puffs while I breathed deeply and looked around.

It was a sunny day and the completely different perspective of being in the lake at eye level with the water took me by surprise. I could see ducks and a swan swimming nearby and clouds rushing by overhead, their reflections mirrored in the smooth water of the lake. It was great and I knew right there and then that lake swimming was already a million times more fun than the chlorine-, pensioner- and piss-filled swimming pool.

I took my time and swam to the first buoy where the others were waiting for me. We floated on our backs for a bit and then swam for a bit more. I did the whole lap like this with lots of little breaks and it felt very liberating to pretty much swim where I liked, without the constraints of a lane to swim in and others tapping at your feet and pushing you along.

As we changed into our cycling gear I felt exhilarated, if a little seasick. In my head I knew that I had quietly achieved something significant that morning amongst all those real triathletes and I liked it. All I needed now was to wait for my testicles to descend again.

In the Presence of Ironmen

THE TRAINING was moving along to plan but I couldn't shake the feeling that it was harder than it should have been at this easy stage; I felt like I was already struggling to progress. My old lazy genes were creeping back and I'd even skipped a couple of sessions. My heart rate was through the roof and I was sweating like a horse at the very thought of doing any exercise. I couldn't decide if this was the fact that I was 43 and that's what happens when you become an old git, or if it was the cancer reminding me it was there. Either way, what was I going to do about it now? All I could do was plough on and see what happened. 'Get back in that pool you moaning old sod,' I told myself.

What I needed now was an event in the diary to give me the motivation, or more likely the fear, to knuckle down. During the last couple of months all I had found myself thinking about was Ironman and the challenges involved with that. It was definitely a good way to keep my mind occupied and away from the dark stuff and I was constantly studying the Ironman website, reading blogs and magazines and looking at the races to decide in my mind which, if any of them, I might like to do.

There are a few ways you can look at it to help you decide. You can pick on location, maybe somewhere warm and exotic, and combine it with the holiday of a lifetime. Sounds great but warm and exotic could mean a non-wetsuit swim, no chance. You can pick a flat one, which would undoubtedly be an easier race, just to get a medal, or you could pick something more difficult for the challenge. One of the world's most difficult races is the Ironman Wales held in Tenby, Pembrokeshire, on or around the second week in September, and this was the one that I kept coming back to.

The timing of it was tight but doable and the thought of doing a race on home soil felt somehow more authentic and necessary in my book. Researching the race, I quickly learnt the pitfalls of this particular event. It isn't called 'the dragon' for nothing, that's for sure.

It starts with the 2.4-mile sea swim off the town's north beach. The tides there can be against you for large portions and depending on the weather in September, the racers can face big waves and deep swell. The water is cold as well, typically around 16 degrees Celsius, and to cap it all the water can be full of jellyfish, some of which can be as big as dustbin lids.

Transition during a triathlon, i.e. the distance from the swim to the bikes, is usually only a few yards, but Ironman Wales has the longest transition of all, with a steep run on a zigzag footpath up the cliff face into the town, followed by a one kilometre run across town to get to the transition area. This is unique in all the Ironman events and you get no extra time to do it.

The 112-mile bike leg is over the beautiful but hilly Pembrokeshire countryside. The course incorporates over 7,000 feet of climbing, including four extremely difficult climbs and some equally technical descents. Large sections are very exposed and can be subject to severe energy-sapping headwinds.

The run, which is a full marathon, snakes through the town and heads up into a neighbouring village. The run is almost completely up and down hill. No real flat to speak of and very difficult in its own right, let alone as the conclusion to an Ironman. Combine this with the chance of some shockingly cold, windy or wet Welsh weather and you've got one hell of a challenge. It all sounded absolutely delightful.

I know Wales very well; I've been holidaying there since I was a kid. My grandmother was Welsh and came from the Mumbles area of Swansea, so we would always spend some of the summer holiday visiting and exploring the Gower. I've always been drawn back since for the beautiful coastline and countryside. I definitely feel the Welsh blood in me when I am on Welsh soil, which was making Ironman Wales even more of a natural choice. I knew Pembrokeshire reasonably well but also knew the only way to properly experience the county and the Ironman would be to go there and immerse myself in it. To that end, we booked ourselves a cottage for the week before the Ironman to explore the course and see the race first-hand.

Maria had been training with me a lot of the time and it was great to have someone to exercise with. She was as intrigued as I was by the romance of the Ironman and was just as keen to explore the course. We arrived to some glorious weather and the cottage we had booked was a beautiful old farmhouse nestled in the woodland up the hill from the coastal village of Amroth. It would be the perfect place to relax and explore from.

The first thing we said we would do when we got there was go for a sea swim, another first for me. The sea was shimmering and calm as we arrived and I shocked myself by thinking that it looked quite inviting. So we pulled up our wetsuits and in we went. I was shocked again at how even more buoyant I was in my wetsuit in salt water. This felt good, there would definitely be no drowning today. We swam for about 30 minutes, up and down the bay resting on our backs to watch the sea birds diving around us.

The swim was pretty uneventful and turned out to be actually quite pleasant, but as I wobbled up the stone beach to get out, I realised how seasick I was feeling, and I was physically sick in my mouth as I stood up. I felt quite giddy and very nauseous, and realised that I must have drank most of the sea I had been swimming in. My sinuses were streaming from the salt water and my nostrils felt like they were on fire, not quite the success story I would have liked then. Still, nothing a nose plug and better breathing technique wouldn't solve, I thought as I burped my way back to Maria who was impatiently waiting for me on the jetty. She, as usual, seemed to have suffered no ill effects whatsoever and was buzzing from her swim.

The next day we planned our first bike ride out from the cottage. We could pick up the Ironman course just outside the village and ride what is known as the 'big loop' through Saundersfoot and Tenby, then up to Narbeth before circling back to Amroth and the finish.

It was another warm and sunny day as we set off straight into a real knee-trembler of a hill. We both wobbled from side to side as we crawled up it. What followed was an epic 48-mile bike ride that felt well beyond the current capability of either of us. As the ride went on there were some shockingly steep climbs and other long sections of uphill which seemingly never ended. These were then followed by sketchy, steep and twisting downhills which gave little respite from the long climbs and required total concentration to avoid ending up in the bushes.

We also experienced our first coming-together on that bike ride. I had a printed map of the route in my back pocket and as we were descending a gravelly single-track road, I was wondering if the right turn coming up was the one we needed to take. I slowed down to look at the map and my heart sank as I heard the screeching of brakes behind me followed by a high pitched 'whoa whoa whoa!' I knew exactly what was coming and braced for the impact as Maria came clattering into the back of me. I felt my bike pitch up and tip me off over the bars as I was thrown down the road and into a ditch. I turned to see Maria in a heap on the road behind me with one leg still attached to her bike.

I couldn't bloody believe it, my new bike, it had better not be damaged. I leapt up and pulled it out of the ditch to look at it and then suddenly realised my wife was still lying on the road behind me. I put down the bike and helped her get untangled from hers. I have since forgiven myself for the complete lapse in judgement, by putting it all down to the shock of the moment.

We dusted ourselves off. We were both a bit battered but fortunately neither us nor our bikes were badly injured and we could carry on. Maria seemed to have come off worse with a big bruise and nasty gravelly gash on one of her knees. We both blamed each other in the time-honoured fashion of married couples and Maria had a bit of a sulk for 20 minutes before she eventually caught up with me. We had a little hug and got back to business.

A good few hours later we both sat exhausted in the sun on the sea wall back in Amroth licking an ice cream. We were a bit shell-shocked to think that what we had just struggled around wasn't even halfway on the bike course. If I was mad enough to want to do the race, I would have to do what we just did twice and another 20-odd mile loop on top, just for good measure. Good grief.

Looking back at my training diary, I described it as a terrifying c*** of a bike ride. I make no apology for my use of the other c bomb because in the context of a full Ironman, that's exactly what it was.

We gave ourselves the next day off to recover and rode the final part of the course the day after.

We drove out to the village of Lamphey and parked at the village hall, which was the location of one of the Ironman feed stations. The ride that day took us through Pembroke and along the coast passing the Castlemartin military ranges on our way to the beautiful beach at Freshwater West, then on to the remote coastal village of Angle before returning via Pembroke. We took the ride at a more leisurely pace this time and it was a stunning day out, but bugger me was it hilly again. This section is supposed to be 'the flat bit' and once again I had found another new perspective on the difficulty of this race.

The next day we had a relaxing time exploring the local area with my parents who had joined us for the weekend and then it was Saturday evening. The Ironman was the following morning. We had an early night to be up at five o'clock so we could cycle the coast path into Tenby for the start of the swim, which started at seven sharp.

I was, strangely, quite nervous about it that night and barely slept a wink. I'm not sure why this was, but I think I already had the feeling that I wanted to do it and I didn't want to be scared off by the experience. We were both tossing and turning at four, so got up and had a quick breakfast before cycling off in the pitch black of the pre-dawn to get to Tenby.

When we arrived at the North Beach the sun was just coming up. I couldn't believe how many people were out this early in the morning to see the swim start, there were people everywhere. The athletes were in their wetsuits and were making their way down to the beach for the mass start on the sand. You could feel the crackle of excitement in the air and see the nervousness on the faces of the competitors, it was quite a scene. We chained our bikes to a railing and squeezed into the crowd to get a view of the beach. Looking along the clifftops, there wasn't an empty place to stand, there were hundreds of people watching. The cliffs around the beach make it the perfect amphitheatre from which you can see the drama of the entire swim.

What really struck me seeing all the athletes in their wetsuits walking down to the beach was what different shapes and sizes they all were. I somehow expected everyone to be slim and athletic, but there was a full cross section of body types. Some people were shockingly large and I wondered how on earth they would get that much bulk around such a long course. Obviously my perceptions of what it would take to finish one of these races were slightly skewed – if people like this can manage it or at least give it a go, then why couldn't I?

The sea was alarmingly rough that day after being like a mill pond all week. You could see the swell rolling in from the distance, which was resulting in massive waves crashing on to the beach. Those would certainly take some getting through, just to get out into the swell. The thought of having to do that myself was terrifying. It's not like this every year, I told myself.

I could see the athletes down below us on the beach. Around 2,000 men and women crammed together in a roped-off funnel towards the foaming tide line. The professionals were in the water just in front of them. Suddenly the Welsh anthem 'Land of My Fathers' rang out across the bay. I hadn't expected this and the stirring music, accompanied by the Welsh crowd's spontaneous singing, made me shiver with goosebumps. It was already a fantastic occasion and I was now totally intoxicated by it.

The horn blew and there was a sudden stampede towards the water accompanied by a massive cheer from the crowd which rolled around the bay as the loudspeakers boomed 'Ladies and gentlemen, we are racing!'

The professionals disappeared off into the bay at a ridiculous speed towards the first giant orange buoy, which was bobbing wildly in the water what seemed like miles from the shore. The age-group athletes followed. Some were evidently expert swimmers themselves but some clearly not so much. As the foaming thrash of swimmers began to spread out across the bay, I could see a few people already being brought back to the beach by the life guards on their jet skis. Their races were over in a matter of minutes – what could have caused that? A kick to the face in the melee of the mass start, or a panic attack? Who knew? But the drama was unfolding right in front of us and it was very exciting to see.

The swim is two laps of a triangular course with a run up the beach and around a marker before returning to the water for the second lap. This is called an Australian exit and adds to the difficulty. The pros exited the water like missiles and sprinted up the beach before diving straight back into the surf and butterfly stroking their way out through the waves and disappearing into the swell again. They had already started lapping some of the slowest swimmers. The age-groupers were more of a mixed bag, some staggered from the water as if they were drunk. I saw one guy plunge head first into the sand. He was covered in it, a proper mouthful. If it had been his second lap he would have had to go back into the sea to wash it off. He couldn't have got onto his bike in that state.

We watched the first-swim finishers run up the slope and clapped them through town before making our way to the transition area to see them coming out on their bikes. Something you learn quickly about triathlon is there is a certain look and a level of kit required. Triathlon is more of an individual time trial than an out-and-out race. You can't employ drafting tactics like you can in a cycle race, so triathletes love to use all the latest streamlined equipment like tear-drop helmets and time-trial specific bicycles. The front runners roared out of transition tucked tightly into their bicycles and were already riding at full tilt. Their disc wheels made their bikes sound like Star Wars Tie Fighters as they shot past us and out on to the bike course.

We stood with a coffee and cheered the majority of people running in and cycling out of transition before returning to the harbour to watch the last of the swimmers. The cut-off is two hours 20 minutes for the swim, and as we rounded the corner I was shocked to see at least 50 people still in the water. It was coming up to two hours now and some were still only halfway around their second lap. It was heartbreaking to realise that they would never make the cut from that position but were still swimming for it. Some were evidently right on the time limit and the lifeguards in the water on their paddle boards were swimming alongside and encouraging that one last big effort to make it to the line. You could see they were all exhausted – this was the real drama of the race.

We watched as the time limit faded with the last hopes of those still bobbing in the ridiculously rough seas before heading back to the cottage for a cooked brunch with my parents. The intention was to return to Tenby later in the day to see the marathon unfold. As we made our way across town, I noticed a few dejected people in wetsuits walking around with their families, some of them in tears. For whatever reason, their races had ended, it must have been crushingly disappointing to be out so early in the day. Seeing them so distraught, you began to realise just how high the stakes were if you chose to put yourself in that position. The risk of failure is very real when weighed against the level of commitment you need to just get yourself to that start line. It's impressive and humbling in equal measure.

That evening, as darkness drew in, we were back in Tenby, the crowds were again unbelievable around the town and there was a real party atmosphere. Some runners were already being cheered over the finish line to shouts of 'YOU ARE AN IRONMAN', but others in the growing darkness elsewhere in the town were locked in a desperate battle to just keep putting one foot in front of the other with the prospect of another five hours of agony to go before their moment on the red carpet.

I was intrigued by these people the most, because I would certainly be one of them. If I was here next year this is where I would be and probably dealing with other painful side-effects from my treatment on top. I needed to see what the business end of this race was like for the ordinary people like me and I wasn't disappointed. The narrow streets of Tenby meant that you were within touching distance of the athletes as they ran past. I was shocked by the smell of it, for one thing. I don't know what I was expecting but the whole experience was a very visceral one. It was seven in the evening and these people had been going for 12 hours straight – some would still have five more to go. You experienced their agonies with all your senses. The sight of the thick white salt stains on their tri suits really struck me. That was a real visual indicator of what they had been putting their bodies through that day as they moved forward.

As the crowds thinned into the night, those athletes left were the real heroes who painfully shuffled past us and off again into the gloom. They were lost in their own personal worlds of pain and determination. Shouts of encouragement clearly gave some a little boost and a smile, others didn't even seem to acknowledge that there was anybody else around as they ploughed on. Some were clearly running with painful injuries that they were wrestling with through gritted teeth.

The finish line was a floodlit carnival and was crowded right up until the last finishers at midnight. It was very emotional seeing all the smiles and hugs from family and friends as the finishers came up that red carpet to the cheers of the crowds and the congratulations of the race compères. It was clear to see how hard they had worked and what it meant to them to hear those four magical words 'YOU ARE AN IRONMAN'.

I was a bit overcome by it all and had to turn away and hide a few tears from Maria and my parents. In a single moment under those lights and amongst that crowd I understood what I needed to do to fight the cancer. I was going to be a Welsh Ironman.

I knew right then that this race would be the metaphor for my journey that coming year. I had a mountain to climb just as these ordinary people had done and that red carpet right there would be my summit. An overwhelming desire to live and fight swept over me as each subsequent Ironman came over the finish line. If I crossed that line I'd win. I will have beaten the cancer, and even if it came back and got me later, I had still won.

I didn't even know for sure if I was going to be alive that time next year or the toll the cancer would take on my body, but the very next day when the registration opened for Ironman Wales 2015 my credit card was out and I was in.

Moviprep and the Snake of Doom

BACK FROM Ironman Wales and filled with an invigorated sense of purpose, I got straight back into the ten-week plan and the wholesale change in my mental attitude towards the exercise was palpable. I felt fitter and stronger and much less inclined to miss training sessions. I knew that the honeymoon period of spending 400-odd quid on the entrance fee wouldn't last forever, so I was determined to make the most of it.

At work I delivered the news to Tom that I'd only gone and done it! I could see his face drop a bit as I told him. He knew how tough Ironman Wales was and I think he was hoping to negotiate another half-distance race or at least another warmer, more pleasant Ironman location for our first race. All this chatter was history now though, I had pulled the trigger on Wales and the poor bugger didn't really have much choice but to follow suit. I told him to get his arse in gear and get it booked.

My operation was originally pencilled in for when we returned from our holiday but this had long since been cancelled. I had been contacted by the Basingstoke and North Hampshire Hospital and they wanted me to see a Mr Mohamed for a consultation on 6 October. It appeared that the situation was more complicated than first suspected but I was still required to have the pre-planned colonoscopy and would be sent for yet another scan prior to that meeting.

I was finding the prospect of another scan a little disturbing, not the procedure itself as this was pretty routine but the implications of needing another one. It surely meant that they suspected a spread of the disease or at the very least they wanted to rule it out. My Google research into appendix cancer was telling me that if they had removed my appendix then hopefully they had removed the cancer. This was my best case outcome at present and I was hanging on to that theory for now, but reading between the lines of the consultants' letters they were perhaps telling me something more sinister was going on without implicitly saying it. I was starting to get used to all the guarded doctor speak but it was very difficult not to interpret it badly.

What was very clear though was that further testing and a visit to a specialist consultant suggested a serious situation. All a bit worrying but once again without details what can you do about it? I knew my calm veneer was starting to peel back at the edges and I didn't want to dwell on it too much for fear of a snowballing effect rolling uncontrollably away from me and taking all my coping strategies with it, so for now it was back to the exercise, repeating the mantras and sitting tight.

The dreaded day had finally arrived for the colonoscopy and I wasn't looking forward to it as I knew it would be uncomfortable. Some men get funny about the thought of other men touching their bums but I can honestly say that I wasn't that bothered. I'd already had more fingers up my bum this year than the whole of my life, so I wasn't clenched too tightly at the thought of it.

I had been provided with a box of medicine called Moviprep to cleanse my bowel the day before the procedure. It was necessary to take it so that the doctor performing the procedure could get a good unobstructed look at the inside of my large intestine and get a run at going all the way around without it being backed up like a motorway rush hour.

I was told that due to the very effective nature of the medicine I should under no circumstances attempt to go to work the day I was taking it. I sensibly took that advice and spent the day at home sporting some loose-fitting jogging bottoms and ensured that I remained within a short waddle from the toilet at all times. I had to drink one litre of Moviprep at midday and another at around six in the evening. I had read that some people found it beneficial to make it up earlier and chill it in the fridge to make it more palatable. I had to drink each litre as quickly as possible if I could, but at least within the hour.

Lunchtime came and I was stood at the kitchen sink with my Pyrex measuring jug and tore the sachet with my teeth to open it. A sherbet lemony waft of powder came up out of the packet and I thought that it didn't seem that bad. As I mixed it into the water, I could see that it was quite thick as it dissolved. I had to stir it for quite a time for all the powder to disappear from the bottom of the jug and I was then left with a litre of cloudy lemon squash-smelling and slightly oily-looking liquid. My plan was to get it down me in four manageable glasses and do it as quickly as I could to get it out of the way.

I took my first big glug and instantly started to shudder. My gag reflex was making the back of my throat wobble as I forcefully swallowed it down – it was disgusting. In fact, it was one of the most hideous things I'd ever drunk. The lemon flavour was clearly there to mask the foul-tasting medicine but why bother. It tasted like cheap lemon squash made up with particularly briny seawater and then mixed with a few tablespoons of olive oil to make it slip down, the oily texture making it stick to my mouth. Realising how bad it was going to be, I went for it and did the rest of the glass in one go to finish it.

I coughed, shuddered and poured another glass and downed that as well. This made me retch, so I rinsed my mouth with some clean water and gave it ten minutes before returning to finish the rest. By the last mouthful my eyes were running and I was sweating and gagging, but I'd got through it and I made up the next litre for later. This one was definitely going in the fridge – maybe I could sip it over ice and pretend it was a cheap margarita.

The downstairs toilet had already been prepared with baby wipes, Vaseline and a spare toilet roll so all that was left to do was settle down and watch some daytime television until it was time to go. It was at least

30 minutes before the first gurgling noises started and I was beginning to wonder if it was working. These initial gurgles were quickly replaced by growls and howls which sounded like agitated jungle animals and were accompanied by strong cramping, squeezing and weird vibrating sensations coming from deep inside me.

After ten minutes of this all-consuming sensory spectacular, I was rushing stiff-legged into the toilet. I barely managed to sit myself down before what I can only describe as an explosion occurred beneath me.

I had only just got cleaned up and left the toilet when I was rushing straight back in again. What felt like a gallon of rusty water spiralled out of me into the bowl as I clung to the sides of the toilet seat and clenched my teeth. I had never experienced anything like this before. Where was all this water coming from? I'd only drunk a litre of the stuff.

One hour in and it was still pouring out of me in long toe-curling squirts and only after two hours did it start to slow down. By this point I was exhausted and my only thought was that I've got to do all this again in two hours' time. I wondered if the doctor would recognise what he was looking at the next day, I felt so sore down there. I dabbed on some more cream and went for a lie down.

Maria came home from work and found me laid out like a wounded animal on the sofa. She laughed loudly as I told her what had been happening and she went off to make her dinner, not wanting me anywhere near the cooking that day for obvious reasons. I, on the other hand, was nil by mouth and starving. Six o'clock came and I was back in the kitchen breathing deeply and eyeing up my next jug. My tactics didn't change from the first round and 20 miserable minutes later I was finished and back lying on the sofa waiting for the inevitable. It came quicker this time, but was no less of a violent experience. I felt like I was in a scene from *The Exorcist.* There were certainly some demons being exorcised judging by the weird sights that were greeting me from the bottom of the bowl. What the hell was that stuff, I swear I saw a small toy soldier I must have swallowed when I was about five.

Another two emotional and quite frankly painful hours had passed. The flood waters eventually subsided and the damage could be surveyed. Sore wasn't really touching how I was feeling down there and I certainly wasn't relishing the intimate encounter I was due the next day. I staggered from the toilet straight upstairs. I managed a quick shower and fell straight into bed exhausted, what a day that was. They weren't joking when they said don't go to work. I drifted off to sleep plotting how much of the stuff I could get into Tom's Ironman mug without him noticing.

The next day I felt surprisingly sprightly. I guessed this was the euphoric feeling people talk about when they've had a colonic irrigation or an enema in one of those Thai spas. It was either that or a dehydration-induced delirium.

I had to report to the hospital an hour before my appointment and was filling in a questionnaire about my general health as I looked around the waiting area. I was struck by how old everyone else was. I must have been the youngest by at least 20 years that day. One thing we all had in common though was an air of apprehension as our names were called and we disappeared, one by one, behind the curtain never to be seen again.

When my time came to pass through it, I was greeted on the other side by a smiling nurse who gave me a bag for my clothes and a robe to put on. She also passed me a giant pair of paper underpants and helpfully reminded me to put them on with the hole at the back.

I was taken through to the procedure room and greeted by a very cheerful doctor and his equally cheerful nursing assistant. I know they were doing their best to make me feel comfortable but the thick black articulated snake with the camera on the end of it that I saw flexing out of the corner of my eye as I lay down on the bed put a swift end to any thoughts of relaxation I may have been pretending to feel.

I faced away from the doctor and was told to draw my legs up towards my chest and into a foetal position. The nurse was on my side of the table and was telling me to breathe deeply and to try to relax as much as possible. I could see a monitor on the wall in front of me. It flickered into life and as the image focussed it was flashing between a close-up of the doctor's hairy nostrils and the walls of the room before it started snaking its way towards my paper pants.

I felt a cold blob of cream on my backside which I was told was a mild anaesthetic to numb my bum as the camera went in. There was no hanging around after that. I barely felt a thing as the image on the monitor suddenly went dark before flashing a shockingly large close-up of my puckered bumhole and then in an instant started illuminating the inside of my back passage. I was struck by how fascinating it is to see the inside of your own body – as the camera slowly nudged its way inside I could clearly see the shiny pink ridged sides of my bowel covered with a fine layer of mucus. I was surprised how clean it was up there. The Moviprep had certainly done its job as there were only a couple of specks to be seen – how they managed to cling on yesterday I'll never know.

The large intestine goes from your rectum around the outside of your lower abdomen in a kind of square, so the camera has three pretty much 90-degree bends to negotiate. As the camera reached the first of these bends I felt this incredibly deep ache inside my left side. I wasn't expecting it to be that painful. I was informed while reading the pre-procedure paperwork that some discomfort may be experienced but that was a bit of an understatement to say the least. I gave out an involuntary groan and tried to stay relaxed and fight the overwhelming urge I had to leap from the table, certainly not a good move to make at that precise moment. The nurse offered me her hand to hold and I grabbed it and squeezed hard as the pain slowly subsided when the camera made the bend and carried on its journey.

The second bend was negotiated in a similar fashion and we soon reached what was left of the root of my appendix and the end of my large intestine. The doctor explained what he was seeing as he went and I was aware that he was looking for polyps and cancerous growths which may have spread to my bowel. He was particularly interested in the area around where my appendix had been, as this was a likely spot for any cancer to be seen.

I'm no expert obviously, but I could see it all looked pretty clean in there. My own observations coupled with the positive noises coming over my shoulder from the doctor made me feel good. There certainly wasn't a horror show greeting us up there and that was a big relief. He took a little snip of some skin near my appendix for testing, which I didn't feel at all, and it was done.

He withdrew the camera with what I thought was a bit of indecent haste and it took my breath away as the snake blinked back into the outside world and refocused its eye on the wall behind us. I realised then that I was still holding the nurse's hand and gave it a last little squeeze before thanking her for looking after me.

That was the second time I had grabbed the hand of a nurse during a rough moment – the first was during my drain insertion back in June and it makes me smile to think that a big tough guy like me would get so much comfort from the simple act of holding a stranger's hand. It goes to show you should never turn down any offers of support when the going gets tough.

The whole colonoscopy journey was an experience for sure, but it was ultimately a positive one for me. Although the results of the examination would need to be read by Dr Mohamed in conjunction with my scans and blood results, I already knew that the inside of my bowels appeared to be cancer free; it was just for Mr Mohamed to tell me about the outsides of them now and that day was approaching fast.

Pseudo Mix What?

I WOKE up early on 6 October 2014 and took myself straight into the shower. I stood and let the water wash over me as I contemplated the day ahead. This was the day that I would find out what was wrong with me and potentially how long I had left and it felt surreal to be contemplating it. This day had been such a long time coming with so little information that I wasn't getting excited just yet. I felt healthier than I had in years, which made it even more difficult to comprehend that I had a potentially fatal disease hiding away inside me.

What was I expecting from the day? A treatment plan? A timescale? Some details about the disease itself? Some sort of view on life expectancy? Fuck, that one really dug deep. Will I be fighting a painful battle in the husk of my previous self just to stay alive a bit longer or will I get lucky and live a long and happy life after my treatment? Who knew?

Maria and I sat and had a pretty tasteless breakfast and then drove in near silence to the hospital. We were both preoccupied with our own thoughts and worried about what questions we should ask when we got there. This time I did have a list written down, unlike before, and I was determined to come out with at least some knowledge of my condition, which had really been lacking since my initial diagnosis, that now felt like a lifetime ago.

The waiting area was busy as we were meeting in the outpatients' department but this time we were ushered straight through to the consultant's office on time. Sat behind the desk was Mr Mohamed. He rose to greet us both and introduced himself with a smile. Behind him was one of the specialist cancer nurses. He was a slight, sharply dressed and well-spoken man and appeared quite young in comparison to other consultants I had met previously. In those first moments the impression of him was one of calm confidence and authority, someone you could trust with your life maybe.

We sat and got straight down to business. Mr Mohamed told me that he had studied my scans, bloods and colonoscopy, and my histology showed that I had been diagnosed with a moderately differentiated mucinous adenocarcinoma, a form of Pseudomyxoma Peritonei.

A what? I was in complete information overload already. It was the first time I had heard any terms other than appendix cancer before now – it all sounded so much more serious and it made my head spin. I had to back up and asked for more detail straight away.

He explained that Pseudomyxoma Peritonei is a rare cancerous growth which results in an accumulation of tumour cells within the abdomen and pelvis. It begins when a cancerous growth inside the appendix bursts through the wall of the appendix and spreads mucus-producing tumour cells throughout the surrounding surfaces. As these tumour cells accumulate, the abdominal area becomes swollen with mucus and tumours and over time it results in obstruction of the intestines or the loss of intestinal function. It can lead to poor food intake, malnutrition and eventually life-threatening complications. It is a very rare disease and only effects about two in a million people. Blimey.

Mr Mohamed placed a copy of part of my latest scan against the light board behind him and turned it on. He explained in no uncertain terms that I would need a substantial operation to treat the disease. He referred to the scan and pointed to three areas he believed the cancer had spread into.

My scans showed disease in the right groin area and more disease in the area of my now removed appendix and again in the region of my belly button. There was a risk of spread to the lymph nodes and then other organs, but this could only be determined after the operation when the lymph nodes that are removed can be analysed for the spread of disease.

Mr Mohamed explained that he would remove the right side of my large intestine and join it with my small intestine, strip the right side of my body cavity of its peritoneum or the internal skin of the body cavity and then remove my omentum, which is a fatty skirt on the front of the abdomen. He would then look for further disease inside my body cavity. He needed to search carefully for the tumours as they can be very small in comparison to the quantities of mucus that they produce. To prevent the cancer returning, he would wash my abdomen with a warm chemotherapy solution. This is referred to as hyperthermic intraperitoneal chemotherapy or HIPEC. The chemotherapy is heated to 42 degrees Celsius inside the abdominal cavity to increase the penetration of the drugs into any tumour that may have been left behind. If it was appropriate, he would follow up my treatment with more chemotherapy administered in the days following surgery.

He showed me on the scan an area deep in my groin which appeared to show disease near the psoas muscle, meaning that my femoral nerve could be at risk. He warned me that any damage to the femoral nerve could result in a drop foot and the need to wear a leg brace, but this would not be clear until he operated. This news shocked me and was the first time I realised that everything might not actually be alright and I could end up damaged for life.

There was a chance that I may require a temporary ileostomy resulting in the need for a colostomy bag, but again this could only be determined during the surgery. The only real way to assess the damage was to open me up and deal with what was found as not all the tumours would necessarily show up on the scans. The bottom line was I would walk into the surgery not knowing what my outcome would be until I woke up on the other side.

The surgery would last for about eight hours and was a serious medical procedure which would require a three-week stay in hospital to recover. Occasionally people don't survive surgery but this was rare and I was young and fit, so he saw no reason for me not to make a full recovery.

All these details were washing over me in sickly tidal waves. What was I hearing? This was serious shit and so much more than I could have possibly imagined. I was undoubtedly shell-shocked and still trying to come to terms with what I was being told.

I asked him if he felt I could still do an Ironman the following September. He didn't even know what one was, and when I explained he smiled and said they don't call it the 'Mother of all Surgery' for nothing. There may also be a requirement to have follow-up chemotherapy but this would only become clear after the operation. This, of course, would affect any training on top of coping with the physical recovery from such an invasive procedure. He did a good job of avoiding answering that one.

In just two months I'd gone from requiring a planned keyhole procedure with my original consultant to this. It was a sobering thought and one which sent my head into a spin.

I was still clinging to the Ironman as my route through it all. Every detail I was digesting I was putting into context of the event and my training, even as I sat in that consulting room gripping Maria's ever tightening hand. I wasn't going to go to pieces here, I was going to calculate a way through it even with a drop foot and a bag. The cold hard reality was, of course, what the hell did I know? I had no idea what either of those things really meant practically.

Life expectancy never really came up. Maybe I choked and swerved it as I looked down my list of questions, or maybe it was the fact that Mr Mohamed told me that his ultimate aim was to cure me during surgery by removing all of the disease, which gave me some comfort for the future. One thing was for sure, I didn't come out of that room thinking I was going to be dying anytime soon, well apart from possibly on the operating table, but that was something I couldn't influence.

The operation was booked for Thursday, 20 November, so there was a good chance I would be home for Christmas.

It did concern me that I had waited a long time for this date and treatment plan. Would these delays since my diagnosis make any difference to the outcome? I was assured that although my disease was considered medium grade, it was very slow to spread so it was unlikely that the wait would cause any significant changes in the diagnosis. I would have another scan in the meantime to assess the depth and detail of the tumour in my groin in more detail.

There was a chance he would need to remove my spleen as well, so I was given a referral letter and told to get a long list of jabs from my doctor four weeks before I was admitted.

We then spent some time with the specialist cancer nurse in the next room who provided us with some more leaflets to read and asked us if we had any questions. By that stage our brains had run out of steam and I certainly couldn't think of anything else to ask. She gave us her details in case we had any other questions later.

We walked out of the hospital hand in hand, both in shock and trying to absorb the news. On the one hand it wasn't the hopeless cause some get dealt, but on the other was a monster of an operation and there was still a massive uncertainty for what lay ahead of us. We couldn't make our minds up if we were feeling relieved or more unsettled by the news. At least we could start to plan and move forward, and I even had a name for my cancer, Pseudomyxoma Peritonei, which in its own way felt good.

One thing was crystal clear – if I thought I needed to be in shape for my treatment before today I was now convinced of it. Bring it on, in six weeks I could get that shit out of me.

The Race for Life

FOLLOWING MY consultation with Mr Mohamed, the time dragged very slowly. For a couple of days I struggled to find the motivation to do much at all. I was still dragging my arse to work, but my mood was very low. We were going through a really lean period and as a specialist team we didn't have a lot to do. I was grateful though, as it gave us time to sit back, drink more tea and talk a lot in the office. The company of friends has always been important to me and we had a good laugh entertaining ourselves every day as we scratched around trying to find things to do.

Tom had entered the Ironman now, which was great news, and we spent far too much time discussing it in far too much length and detail. He reckoned he would beat me and took great delight in describing how he wouldn't gloat too much as he made his victory speech. I was very relaxed about it and enjoyed pointing out to him that it would be a very hollow victory to beat a man ten years his senior with cancer. On the flip side, if he was to lose to a man ten years his senior with cancer, then that would be a very poor show indeed. He couldn't win either way, just how I liked it.

If I needed any confirmation about how serious my operation was going to be then my colleagues' shocked faces when I explained the details told me everything I needed to know. Sometimes it felt like I needed reminding that this was happening to me and not somebody else. Although I knew it was unlikely, there was a small chance I wouldn't come out of that operating theatre alive. If that was going to be the case I only had six weeks left, and six weeks was no time at all.

At best I would wake up from the operation seriously damaged physically and the mountain to climb back to health from that alone would be difficult, let alone the challenge I had set myself to complete an Ironman on top of it.

This was the first time I started to wonder if I was being unrealistic about what I could achieve post-operation. I researched ileostomy and drop foot syndrome and neither filled me with much confidence. If I looked at it from a cup-half-full perspective, they weren't game enders – both could be overcome with difficulty. I wasn't ready to give up on the dream just yet.

I thought about my life a lot in those few days before I dragged myself mentally and physically back to some form of normality. I thought about Maria and it broke my heart to think of her mourning me. I wanted her to be happy more than anything and was gutted she was having to go through this. I had these morbid fantasies where I could see her sat crying at the crematorium. They were horrible thoughts.

I have very few regrets in my life. I have done some truly wonderful things and had some great adventures along the way. I believed if the time came to say goodbye I could do it with dignity and respect for myself and my family, and one thing that frightened me more than anything else was going out kicking, screaming and frightened. I was digging deep into my reserves already but resolved to keep it together for my family and friends. I wasn't kidding myself though, I hadn't been told I was dying and if that time came then I knew that would be when the real test would begin. I wanted people to be inspired by the way I handled my illness and, heaven forbid, my death. I didn't want people to see me scared and that fear then frightening them. I was getting used to the idea of death being around but that didn't mean that other people were.

If I was to die on the operating table it would happen on 20 November 2014. There really is nothing like a deadline to get your head in order and your arse in gear. To help me deal with it, I spent a lot of time reflecting on what it meant to be alive – the being dead bit was more difficult to address but they do go hand in hand. But thinking about living is clearly the more appealing of the two to fill your head with.

I began to see that life is very precious and it's easy to walk through it taking it for granted. I started to notice all the people around me who were stuck in shit jobs and relationships that were making them unhappy. It's easily said, but life is far too short to waste, and ignoring living makes the shock of death even harder when you have to address it.

The old cliché goes 'we are all going to die one day', but who truly believes that? You might die regretting what you did in life but you're much more likely to regret the things you didn't do. The biggest waste of all is living thinking it will all last forever.

I am not a religious person but I can see the attraction of religion to people at times like these. I know in my heart that when death comes to me it will be a black nothingness, like a deep sleep. So once it's done there will be nothing to fear from death itself. It's the fear of leaving everything you love that breaks your heart and frightens you.

I came to believe that knowing I might die on a certain date is a privilege in a funny sort of way. Better that than getting run over by a bus without the chance to look the people you love in the eye and tell them you love them. Better that than being snatched away with no will written or arrangements made for the people you love. I had six weeks to do all these things so I set about doing it. I wanted to go into that operation knowing my shit was in order. I could then stride through those swing doors to the operating theatre with my gown flapping behind me confident that if I didn't come out the other side I could rest happy knowing that I had done all the things I wanted to.

So we set about sorting out our final will and testaments, something surprisingly easily done and equally easily put off. I also took some time out to write a funeral plan with music and a few words which I sealed up and passed to Maria in an envelope marked dramatically 'To be opened in the event of my death'. All these preparations felt good and helped a great deal to settle my nerves.

A few days after the consultation we were off to Mallorca for a last-minute week in the sun. It was a ridiculously cheap all-inclusive resort which was barely a third full and the weather was in the mid-20s all week with lovely clear blue skies. We stayed in Port de Pollenca, a beautiful seaside port on the north of the island and picked it because it was where Tom had completed his now mythical Ironman 70.3 the year before. We hired some good quality racing bikes and took in some of the famous Mallorcan climbs. The whole week was great and I felt in good shape; the climbs were hard and hot but we managed them with some degree of dignity. We cycled in the morning and sunbathed by a ridiculously cold swimming pool in the afternoon.

All-inclusive holidays have their own rhythm that is very easy to slip into. Cocktails in the afternoon, pre-dinner drinks before the all-you-can-eat buffet, then settling down to the crappy entertainment in the bar surrounded by leathery chain-smoking cockney pensioners in the evening. The cancer was put to the back of our minds and we just enjoyed each other's company. We had a great time and both came back relaxed, tanned and feeling fit.

My next delightful outing when we got back was for the jabs I needed in case my spleen was removed during the operation. I was due to have injections for meningitis B and C, pneumococcal and flu. Apparently if your spleen is removed, it affects your resistance to disease and some people have to remain on low level antibiotics for the rest of their lives. I really hoped I wasn't going to have to be one of them.

I had an early-bird appointment with the nurse at my doctor's surgery and all four injections were administered that day. Each one had its own little package and the vials and needles varied massively as well. I went for all four in my arms after being given the choice of locations as my backside had been exposed to far too many medical practitioners recently. Needless to say, they varied in pain levels from mildly irritating to being injected with acid.

I could barely lift my arms as I left the surgery, which made a good excuse to skip my scheduled swim session. I was still surprisingly nervous each time I went to the pool, despite all the swimming I had been doing recently.

That week I was marking time waiting excitedly for the weekend to come. I was squeezing in a last trip away, mountain biking in Wales with two of my best friends before my operation. We were travelling down to South Wales early on the Friday morning and would spend the day in the Afan Forest with its trails, hopefully, all to ourselves and then a bit more biking on Saturday before driving into Cardiff for a big Saturday night out.

I was getting worried though as I'd developed a pain in the back of my right leg which wasn't going away. It was a deep dull ache through my butt cheek right down my leg and into my foot and I just couldn't get rid of it. At night I struggled to get comfortable and was rolling around stretching and bending trying to find some relief. Being kept awake at night was doing me no favours as it allowed my mind to dwell on things as I lay there and I wondered if the pain was due to the cancer. The doctors told me about the possible nerve damage in my leg and I thought how miserable it would be if this was something I'd have to put up with for the rest of my life. A bit of Googling convinced me that it was a bout of sciatica brought on by all the cycling I had been doing. I tried to stretch it out, hoping it would be gone before the weekend.

Friday came but the sciatica was still lingering as we loaded up the car and went off. I sat bolt upright in the back for the whole journey and much to my relief when we got out at the other end it was gone – I couldn't believe it. We kitted up in the mist and rode off for a great day cycling a tough circuit called The Wall. As the name suggests there was going to be a lot of off-road climbing right from the start and the boys raced off as soon as we turned on to the first uphill section.

Straight away I was puffing and it was difficult to find grip with my tyres on the wet stony trail. I was weaving around all over the path and gutted that I was struggling so badly. I assumed that all the exercise I'd been doing would have had at least some noticeable impact on my fitness. My mates were gym bunnies and I knew for sure that they hadn't done the cardio work I had done recently. As I emerged firmly in last place on to the disused railway line at the end of that first section, I saw the two of them slumped over their handlebars, coughing and wheezing. They both looked decidedly pale and I realised with relief that it was bravado that had overcome them and they had started racing each other right from the off. After that I was pleased to see I had the making of them as they huffed and puffed around the valley. I could feel that I was stronger and this was good. My exercise was paying off after all and the cancer didn't appear to be affecting my performance.

We were due to have a second ride out on the Saturday but the Welsh weather was atrocious and as we were really feeling the effects of the epic ride the day before and the beers from that evening, we gave it a miss. Lots of coffee and a big fried breakfast was in order, followed by a slow sightseeing ride into Cardiff. We all agreed we needed to save energy for our big night out.

We had a great time out on the town and got very drunk aided by lots of Red Bull and vodka to keep us awake. Rolling back to the hotel at three in the morning, we talked about the cancer. None of us have ever been good at expressing our emotions, but aided by the alcohol a few tears were shed and some hugs shared. I was bowled over by how upset my best mate Luigi was, he really didn't want to lose me. I realised I had been so wrapped up in it all that I hadn't really considered what I meant to the people who loved me other than my family, and I vowed to not lose sight of that. Driving back the next day in near silence with a dry mouth and a banging headache, I sat staring at the nasty pre-packed egg sandwich and bottle of Lucozade in my lap and reflected on a great weekend. If it was going to be the last one like it, I had no regrets, that was for sure.

The next week I dragged myself back into work and although the laughs were still good, I started to wonder what the hell I was still doing there. If this was the last few weeks I had on this earth then why was I spending them sitting in this dump waiting for five o'clock to come around every day? I told my boss that Friday would be my last day, leaving me just two weeks before my operation. He was great about it; in fact, he said that he was surprised I'd lasted as long as I had. Everyone wished me the best and Tom and the rest of my close team took me for a coffee on my last day and that was it, I packed my bag and left at lunchtime. Although I wasn't leaving the job it felt like a chapter was closing as I got in the car to drive away. I loved working in that team and we'd had some great adventures over the last couple of years. I was sad to see it end.

As a motivation before going into hospital and to keep me training, I entered a cross country race on Dartmoor called the Drogo Ten. It was a very hilly ten-mile fell run through the valleys surrounding Drogo Castle which also happened to be one of Maria's favourite spots in the whole country. We could combine it with a nice few days away as a last-minute treat and spend some time together before I went under the knife.

I'd set a target of two hours for the race which was doable but still a very decent time for me and I would need to train to the distance to achieve it. The problem was that although I was now training at least five times a week following my Iron Fit programme, I wasn't hitting that kind of distance or time on my feet yet. I needed to up my game and set myself a two-week intensive running programme. I ran for an hour at least three times a week in the dark evenings around the town and included plenty of hilly routes to build strength. Two days before we left for Dartmoor, I ran nine hilly miles on a particularly cold and dark evening. I got back and hit the shower pleased with my work, but that evening I crashed into bed early in a shivery mess. Maybe I had overdone it a bit but I knew I had done enough to keep my target in my sights.

We had two nights booked in the spectacular Bovey Castle Hotel on Dartmoor, with its even more spectacular whisky bar and I enjoyed sitting in front of the huge roaring fireplace perusing the leather-bound whisky menu. I felt every bit the country gent and ignoring the eye-watering prices, I was served some very fine whiskys whilst sat in a red leather wing-back chair.

There was, however, some important business to attend to and we moved to a closer and cheaper hotel nearer the race venue. I had an early night and an even earlier breakfast as it was an 8:30am race start and I still had to register in the morning and collect my race number.

We arrived at Drogo Castle and there was a buzz about the place that you only get on race mornings. There were a lot of very fit and very skinny people trotting about. This was no fun run and it seemed to be mostly good-quality club runners in their colourful race vests milling about at the start. I placed myself near the back of the pack for safety and waited for the gun to signal the start.

It was clear that the start was critical for most of the racers in the pack. The Drogo Ten began on the wide road out from the castle before turning right on to a single track footpath which snaked its way down into the valley. If you weren't at the front then you'd be held up in the pack with little opportunity to overtake for a good ten minutes. This naturally resulted in a wild stampede up the road straight from the gun and as we hit the single track I was already puffing like a madman. My training was all heart-rate based and I was training to a 150 to 160 beats a minute maximum. I looked at my watch and it was blinking 185 back at me. I needed to calm down and fast, or my race was going to fade away before it had even started.

Fortunately, the narrow track combined with a steep downhill slowed the pack up and I had time to recover and get into a bit of a rhythm. The line of colourful runners zig-zagged down the hill through the mist and, impossibly, I could already see people ascending the other side of the valley into the distance. As we reached the woods at the bottom of the valley we had to cross a tiny bridge over a fast-running stream. There was a big queue to get over it so I took the opportunity to recover fully. That felt good but glancing at my watch I knew the precious minutes that were ticking away would punish me at the end. I'd have to work a little harder to make up time now.

Although I was only racing myself, I was a little alarmed to see how thin the field had already become as I took my turn to cross over the bridge. In a quick glance behind me I estimated only about 40 puffing red faces left. As I looked ahead, runners were spreading out into the distance up the hill.

A couple of people came past me and I took the decision to run up the other side of the valley to bring some time back. I felt good and I overtook a few who had previously come past me at the bridge, but I knew I couldn't keep it up – my heart rate was through the roof again and I was fading badly. I gasped for breath and started walking as the valley steepened yet again. It was now a case of hands on knees and pressing on as best I could. I crested the hill and began to descend again. My speed picked up and I was again running faster than race pace so making up some good time. I was back in control and felt pretty good.

I was about four miles in when I fell into stride with a woman who must have been in her late 50s. She was in good shape a and wore the vest of a local running club. I made a joke about the hilliness and she asked me where I was from and what I was doing in this obscure little race. I thought for a second whether she'd want to hear my story but sod it, she asked.

I told her that I had a type of bowel cancer and was going into hospital in two days' time for a big operation so this was my last little treat to myself before I went in. She looked shocked and told me how impressive it was that I was doing the event so close to my treatment. She wished me luck and I was a little shocked to feel her pace kick on a bit. She certainly wasn't feeling sorry for me and obviously didn't fancy being beaten by a man with cancer. I considered staying with her but I was still pretty much on track despite the wait at the bridge, and if I pushed on now it could finish me off.

I reached the valley floor and started the turn back towards the castle. Snaking through the valley, the swollen river was bubbling along and was breaking its banks in places. It was very muddy and it was taking a lot of energy to skip around the deep puddles and sticky mud on the path. About 100 metres in front of me I could see a very tall, barrel-chested man trotting along. He was in a moth-eaten race vest and sported an ancient towelling head band wrapped around his greying Bjorn Borg-style mullet. He was huffing and puffing along and I thought out loud, 'Yes, I'll have you.'

What then proceeded must have been the slowest overtake in amateur fell running history. It took a good ten minutes for me to catch him up and then another awkward ten minutes of running alongside each other without acknowledging each other's presence. I could feel him quickening every now and again to try to open a gap, but I stuck doggedly with him. Eventually a gap the thickness of a cigarette paper opened up between us and it seemed to do the trick. I had finally broken this 60-something fat man and was triumphantly starting to pull away in excruciating slow motion.

It was on that muddy path in the middle of Dartmoor that I discovered a competitive spirit in me which had never previously come to light. I was tasting racing for the first time as opposed to just taking part and it felt good. I realised that being preoccupied with only finishing allows a laziness to creep into your performances because as long as you can finish you don't really need to try any harder. Who cares when you always get a medal and the plaudits for finishing? No one was expecting you to be on the podium anyway. It was a surprisingly good feeling to be pitting myself against someone else and actually winning.

This race was now hotting up but so was my race for life and I didn't want to lose that one, even to a 60-year-old fat man with bad hair. By channelling a bit of competitiveness, even if it was just with myself, I could push myself on that little bit harder.

My heart rate was now plateauing at 168 and I could barely breathe, but in my little micro race through the valley I had made up the time I needed to get in under the two-hour mark. I crossed back over the stream and knew it was going to be one last exhausting push back up the valley to the finish. I turned a tight left off the wide track and into an immediately steep ascent. This one was seriously steep and there would be no one running up here. The hands were back on the knees and I was pushing through the thighs and powering up as quickly as I could.

Ten minutes into the ascent and my thighs were screaming but I had to keep pushing on. I had two others for company now and I allowed them to pass so I could use them for pacing to make it to the top of the climb in good time. Suddenly the path dipped down in a sweeping curve, skirting the valley before disappearing back into the trees. I was still walking as I began the descent and I knew I should have been running, so when an old man in his 80s with a walking stick and flat cap shouted at me to 'Get a move on you lazy git!' I knew he was right. My two hours was again in jeopardy and so close to the finish as well.

I opened up the burning legs and tried to relax my breathing. There were more people cheering me now as the path took another alarmingly steep rise upwards. I knew I must be nearing the finish so I dug in and found some energy to maintain my pace up the incline and, what felt like an age later, I popped out from the trees and the finish line appeared through the mist. I powered on and spotted Maria jumping up and down at the side of the finish area, so I sprinted the last 200 metres across the grass to the finish line, which in true low-key fell running style was a small hand-painted sign on a stick saying FINISH. I was elated to have completed it and grasping at my wrist to stop my watch I could see I had finished in one hour and 58 minutes.

Get in! I was well chuffed. Maria came over and gave me an outstretched hug. I was filthy, stinky and steaming like a racehorse in the cold, damp winter air. I collected a race t-shirt – this wasn't the kind of race where they handed out medals unless you had won.

We went for tea and cake in the National Trust shop on site and I reflected on the last few months. In a funny way we had been freed up by the cancer to do some fantastic things which we would not normally have spent the money to do. I felt good and optimistic for the future. I had done what I set out to do, which was to get fit for the operation. Sat in that steamy, overpriced café, I don't think I could have done any more, so I sat back to enjoy my coffee and Victoria sponge and it tasted great.

That evening back at the hotel we had dinner with a young couple who had just got engaged that day. When the hosts retired to their part of the building, they left the four of us in this big old stone country house in the middle of Dartmoor with the winter wind howling outside. We threw another log on the fire in the snug and got a bit drunk at the honesty bar. It was a great end to a brilliant weekend.

We drove back on the Monday morning after breakfast and I packed my hospital bag. Tomorrow would be the start of another big adventure, although I doubted that there would be so many laughs this time around.

The Mother of all Surgery

IT WAS a pleasant surprise to find myself in a private room when I checked myself in at the Basingstoke and North Hampshire Hospital, and I even had my own little en-suite as well. At least I should be able to get some sleep in here away from the main part of the ward.What wasn't quite so pleasant was the fact that it was 2:30 in the afternoon and I was already nil by mouth. I had the entire next day to get through before my operation, which was scheduled for an early start at 7:30 the day after that. I could literally wet my mouth if it felt dry and that was all, and I was grateful that we'd had a decent brunch before we left home despite not feeling that hungry.

I cracked open the window a little as it must have been about 30 degrees Celsius in the hospital. A fresh breeze blew through it which, despite being the end of November, felt good. Why is it that hospitals are always so bloody hot? I suppose it's all the old people in their pyjamas who must feel the cold. I, on the other hand, was not one of those just yet and was soaking my t-shirt in sweat just lying on my plastic-coated mattress as I sat back and tried to relax. I had brought some comics, magazines and books to keep me occupied. I was watching and reading *The Walking Dead* at the time and had the latest season's DVD to watch on the laptop so I wasn't going to get too bored. If I did I could always count the zombies I saw shuffling around the corridors of the hospital.

Maria went off in search of the accommodation she had been provided in the staff quarters for the duration of my stay. This was perfect as she could remain nearby and maybe even get some work done remotely on her laptop. The rest of that afternoon was taken up with admin, blood tests and introductions to the specialist teams. It was all very relaxed at that stage.

I weighed myself before we had left for the hospital to give myself a bit of a benchmark for where I was before the treatment started. That morning I weighed myself in at 88 kilograms with 26 per cent body fat, nine per cent visceral fat and a body mass index of 25.6. I was a bit shocked it was that high and it looked like I had put on a couple of kilos in the preceding weekends of living it up, despite all the physical activity. I blamed the inaccuracy of the scales we had at home, but at the hospital I weighed in at a healthy or hefty 88.6 kilograms on their clearly more scientific scales. I joked with the nurse that if nothing else it would be good to lose a few pounds whilst I'm here. She laughed and told me that there was a very high likelihood of that happening.

That certainly wouldn't harm my Ironman training as I did appear to be packing a little bit too much excess baggage.

I met my consultant, Mr Mohamed, and his consultant surgeon, Mr Dayal, again that afternoon as they did their ward rounds. They explained that my second scan had been reviewed and showed no further discernible spread of the disease from the first. This was very good news and meant that my wait for surgery had not, on the face of it, harmed my chances of a good recovery at all. They reiterated, however, that they would only know the full extent of the disease once they opened me up. The previously explained risks of nerve damage in my leg and the potential for an ileostomy remained very real threats.

The operation was anticipated to last between seven and nine hours. They would open me up with a full-length cut down my abdomen and then inspect my entire bowel and cavity for signs of disease. They would remove all the disease that they safely could and then remove the full right-hand side of my large intestine and my omentum. They would follow this up by scraping away my peritoneum, which is the internal skin that lines the body cavity and is where the cancer likes to bed itself.

They would then fill my body cavity with the HIPEC chemotherapy for about one and a half hours and rock me from side to side to ensure that it fully contacts all my organs. After that they would insert some drains and stitch me back up.

You can listen to all this information but it is very difficult to fully comprehend what it really means, as it's so far outside your usual realms of understanding. I had already resigned myself to the ride long ago and would deal with each part of the journey as I found it. There was nothing more I could do to prepare and I had no idea of the freight train that was about to hit me; they don't call it the Mother of all Surgery for nothing.

Lymph nodes would be removed during the operation and sent for analysis. If these contained cancerous cells then that would indicate that it was spreading to other parts of my body and would determine whether I required further systemic chemotherapy in the future. The hope was that I wouldn't as I couldn't see rounds of chemotherapy doing my training schedule any favours, but all I could do was keep my fingers crossed.

My hopes of a decent night's sleep didn't come through for me as a procession of nurses marched up and down the corridor and a constant high-pitched beeping in the distance wormed its way into my ears and kept me awake. Lying there with very little to do other than listen to my tummy rumbling gave me plenty of time to reflect.

I was happy and knew I was in the right place. I had done all I could to be fit and healthy for the operation. I had no real regrets in my life and my admin was all sorted. I just needed to relax and let myself be looked after for the next few weeks.

The next morning was a quiet one and I managed to doze off for a bit as Maria tapped away on her laptop in the chair next to me. It got to lunchtime and the nurse came in with a little treat for me – I had to drink two litres of it over the next couple of hours. Yep, you guessed it, the dreaded bowel prep was back, but at least it was going to give me something to do for the rest of the afternoon and evening.

The daily rounds of blood tests started that day as well. The phlebotomy nurses visited me pretty much every day I was in hospital and with each visit they took away in little glass vials what felt like the majority of my blood. I affectionately nicknamed them the vampires.

I also had to sign the disclaimers about subjecting myself to such an intrusive operation. It seems a bit odd and sad that you need to go through what is, in effect, a legal process to disclaim the liability for your life, but it needed to be done and I signed without hesitation. This operation was going to save my life and hopefully allow me to live to a ripe old age, so there was no way I wasn't grasping that opportunity with both hands as without it I was staring at a slow and painful decline that could take who knows how long. It would be unlikely that I'd be drawing a pension without it and that wasn't something I was willing to consider.

As an additional distraction that afternoon I was visited by the stoma nurse. She had the difficult job of explaining the process involved and the equipment associated with a stoma to people like me who really didn't want to be hearing it. She lay out on the bed all the parts of the kit and explained it all in detail.

Although it wasn't clear whether I'd need one, it was important to be exposed to it so the shock wasn't too bad when I woke up. In addition to this she had to mark where my stoma would pop out. I lifted my t-shirt and we discussed where my belt would naturally sit. She then drew a small circle in felt tip on my stomach.

After she left I pulled up my t-shirt to sneak another look at the mark. It was only a small felt tip circle but the implications were a lot more frightening. I think for the first time looking at that mark, I truly accepted what was happening to me, as up until then I had been in my old protective bubble of looking on at what was happening as if I was watching someone else on the television.

This black circle was very real and it was drawn on me. In just 24 hours' time I could be looking at a pink ring of bowel poking out where that circle was. It represented a manifestation of all the fears I had associated with my treatment but not really processed fully and it also reminded me that whatever the outcome in the morning, my life was unlikely to be the same again.

To say I was busy for the rest of the afternoon and evening dealing with the effects of the bowel prep was an understatement. I now understood why I was given a room with an en-suite only a metre from my bed – any further away and there definitely would have been trouble.

Come nine o'clock that evening, as I gingerly dabbed at my burning backside for the last time, I thought I should probably turn in for the night. Maria had returned to her room and was coming back at about 6:30 in the morning to spend some time with me before I went down to theatre. It was all starting to feel very real and very close now.

I looked across the room to my surgical gown and compression stockings folded up neatly on my chair ready for the morning. The nurse would be up for me at about 7:20 to take me down. I elected to walk the corridor to the operating theatre which was located on the same floor as the ward, about a two-minute walk away, as in a weird way it seemed that walking towards your fate was the dignified thing to do. I wasn't sick or overcome with fear, so I didn't need wheeling there, that was for sure.

That evening lying in my darkened room I thought about life, Maria and the next three weeks in hospital. I wondered what the pain would be like and how I would deal with it. I was assuming that I had the luxury of being alive in 18 hours' time and if I wasn't, then I wouldn't know any more about it after the anaesthetist's table so that wasn't worth worrying about. I thought about what I would say to Maria in the morning.

I lay staring at the ceiling for most of the night. It was a good job I was being kept in an induced coma after the operation as I was knackered by the morning. I must have slept at some point, but I woke up around 5:00 and lay quietly waiting until about 6:00 when, unable to just lie there any longer, I got up and took a long, hot shower. The warm water ran over me and I closed my eyes and took some deep breaths to help me relax. I told myself that I'd got this and, feeling surprisingly calm and collected, I dressed for surgery.

Maria came up and we had about 45 minutes before I had to go down. We just sat on the bed quietly and had a bit of a cuddle. She was tearful and I told her that she shouldn't worry and I would be fine. Of course she was going to worry and how the hell did I know what was going to happen, but it felt the right thing to say and, besides, I did genuinely believe it.

It all still felt like a bit of a dream but that all changed at 7:20 on the dot when there was a knock on my room door. Goosebumps erupted all over me as the theatre nurse poked her head around the door and asked if I was ready to go down.

I took a deep breath and smiled back. 'I'm ready,' I said cheerfully.

'Ok then, let's go do this!' was her equally cheerful response.

Maria walked with me hand in hand as far as she was allowed, which was right up to the swing doors into the surgical corridor. This was it then, I hugged her and kissed her hard. I told her that I loved her and would see her on the other side. I looked her in the eyes and smiled then turned and walked through. She was crying. I looked back and we waved to each other as the doors swung shut and she was gone. I took a deep breath. All that was left now was to go through another set of swing doors and into the anaesthetist's area.

A sudden sickly wave of fear washed over me and I thought to myself that I could still escape, but then imagined the undignified scene of me running screaming back through the hospital past an open-mouthed Maria with my gown flapping behind me and decided it would be better all round to just take a deep breath, keep calm and carry on.

The anaesthetist was cheerful as always and within no time at all a cannula was in my arm and I was on the bed lying back and counting down from ten to one. I lay my head back and watched as the milky anaesthetic pumped down the clear tube towards my arm. Seconds after it had disappeared into the cannula there was the familiar tang of metal in my mouth and the world started to close in around me. I closed my eyes and that was that, I was out before I got to five.

Wakey Wakey

THE NEXT thing I remembered was waking up in intensive care. I say waking up, but I was woken up by the horrible sound of someone coughing and gagging loudly somewhere in the room. As I slowly regained my senses, I could hear a muffled voice somewhere in the distance saying, 'Time to wake up Paul, there's a good lad, come on, that's it, well done.' I then had a sudden shocking awakening, my eyes popped open and I realised that the gagging was actually coming from me and I couldn't breathe – an intubation tube was being slid out from deep inside my throat and I was retching violently. As the clear plastic pipe pinged out in front of me with a flick of saliva, I coughed and shouted out my first profound waking words: 'Bloody hell!' The nurse laughed and said, 'Welcome back, Paul.'

So there I was, momentarily back in the world of the living. I blinked around the room trying to focus through blurry eyes and then lay back with a groan, closing my eyes again. 'Wake up now Paul, that's it, do you know where you are?' I opened my eyes again and the smiling nurse stood next to me came into better focus. I felt like I was having some kind of out-of-body experience and my head seemed to be bobbing around about a foot above me. I tried to speak but my mouth was as dry as a bone, my tongue felt like it was the size of an orange and was stuck firmly to the inside of my cheek. The nurse gave me a small squirt of water from a straw into my mouth and I rinsed it around.

I gagged again and confirmed with a smile to the nurse that I was indeed still alive. She told me to take it easy and my family would be in to see me in a bit.

When I say that it was the first thing I remembered, that isn't exactly true. I had come out of theatre at about four in the afternoon and had been kept sedated and intubated until I was woken up at about ten the following morning, and apparently during that time the intensive care nurse had told Maria that I kept fighting the anaesthetic and was quite restless despite being heavily sedated.

I remember being in some strange dreamy place where my body felt paralysed but my mind was being prodded awake every few moments. I was constantly on the verge of sleep but I could hear people's voices around me and the beeping of hospital equipment. I remember that the constant sound of the intubation machine rising and falling with loud shushing air noises was annoying but I'd fall asleep and forget, only to be aware of it again a few moments later.

I remember hearing my family's voices around me whilst I was sedated. At one point I could feel Maria's face very close to mine as she told me how proud she was of me and how much she loved me. I could feel people holding my hand but it felt like my arms were a mile long and my fingers were way off into the distance. I tried to squeeze back but between my waking moments and falling under again, I wasn't sure what I was doing. It was like groundhog day every 30 seconds as I drifted in and out of consciousness.

But there I was all the same, still alive and lying propped against my pillow. I looked around the room. The nurses were at their station opposite me and I appeared to be in a small ward of three beds lined against the wall with a huge array of monitoring equipment around them. The machines around me were constantly whirring and beeping, and I could see my heart rate blipping away on a monitor to my right.

It took me a few moments to get my senses back and remember what the hell I was doing there and that I'd actually just had a major operation, so it was time to take stock. How did I feel? Well, I felt like I had been hit by a train. A dull painful ache was radiating up from my abdomen and it pretty much reached every part of my body. I gingerly lifted the blue hospital blanket that was covering me and pulled up my gown to take a look at the damage. The pen circle was still visible under a stain of brown iodine and remained, thankfully, unused. I lay back again and lowered the covers. Thank fuck for that, the rest of whatever was happening down there could wait for a bit. In that moment it felt like I'd dodged a bullet and although I'd convinced myself before the operation that I could have taken a stoma in my stride, I was mightily relieved I didn't have to test that theory.

The doors to the intensive care unit swung open and I looked up to see a smiling Maria rushing through them towards me. Relief and exhaustion was etched all over her pale face and I knew that the last 30-odd hours must have been a living hell for her as she waited for news about me. She hugged me hard and it made me wince but I didn't care, I was pleased to see her even if my thoughts were still preoccupied.

'How's my leg?' Were the first romantic words I said to her. She told me that there was no nerve damage and the operation went very well. I couldn't believe it. I was secretly convinced that one of those two horrors would have materialised and to hear that neither had happened felt like I had won the lottery and there was nothing more to do than simply leap out of bed and do a quick jig. If only it was all that easy.

On the end of my legs were these blow-up boot contraptions which inflated every 30 seconds or so to help prevent deep vein thrombosis. I'm quite tall and had slid down the bed during the night so my feet were pressing against the footboard. Every time the boots inflated they sent a jolt up my legs which shook my whole body. My left leg was really sore from all this banging, so I asked for the nurse who came and took the footboard away and the relief was instant.

I realised that it must have been those bloody inflatable boots which had kept shaking me awake every 30 seconds throughout my time in intensive care. No wonder I was so knackered from battling the anaesthetic.

Maria has since confessed that she had noticed the boots were causing me to rock against the footboard but in the stress of the moment she didn't think to ask for them to be moved.

Ok, let's have a proper look at what's going on here then. I could see loads of tubes coming out from under the covers which were sticking out of my body in various locations, so I counted them all off.

I had one long bandage down the centre of my abdomen that went from my ribcage literally down to the base of my penis. My incision must be under there, but I would have to wait to get a proper look at that. Although I had given myself a good trim before coming to hospital I could see that my pubic hair had been roughly shaved around the bandage. I knew I'd be grateful to whoever had been given that task when that bandage had to come off.

There were five drains in my abdomen – these were clear plastic tubes stitched crudely into me with thick black thread. They were coming out from both sides of the incision; some were high up and some low down in my groin. They were busy dripping pink fluid into bags suspended from a stand at the side of my bed.

An alarmingly wide catheter came right out of the end of my penis into another bag half-filled with equally disturbing brown piss. I could do with a drink, that was for sure.

A cannula was in my right forearm with two tubes coming from it. One was attached to a fluid bag keeping me hydrated, one drip at a time. The other was being used to give me my cocktail of antibiotics.

A tube was coming out of my right nostril which was being unceremoniously kept in place by a fabric plaster. This was my new best friend: the nasogastric (NG) tube which passed down the back of my throat and into my stomach and it was busy draining a weird bright green liquid into a smaller bag that was pinned on to my gown. Every time I swallowed I could feel it wiggling in my throat. I grew a real love/hate relationship with that tube during my time in hospital. I was told that it was for draining stomach fluid which accumulates at alarming rates when your bowels stop working, as it has nowhere to go other than up and out of your mouth.

A clear plastic pipe was sticking out from between my ribs at the top of my chest on the right side. This was my total parenteral nutrition (TPN) tube and supplied all my nutritional requirements via what looked like a big green bag of premixed energy shake, directly into a vein near my heart.

I also had a small pipe the width of a toilet roll tube stuck up my backside, keeping it open so I didn't have to strain if I needed to go to the toilet. I didn't even know it was there at the time and it would be about a week before it revealed itself. I'll explain that bit of the story later.

I couldn't see it but an epidural in my spine was constantly topping me up with morphine, although at that moment lying there in a lot of pain, I thought that they were being a bit tight with the good stuff.

In all, I counted 11 different pipes and tubes either going in or coming out of me. All of them were sore and added to the overall sensation of discomfort which was smothering me as I lay there trying to keep as still as I could.

I readily admit that I was feeling a bit sorry for myself at that point, something which I vowed not to do before I came into hospital. I was determined not to be the miserable moaning old bugger that got on all the nurses' nerves. I'd experienced enough of those sorts of self-centred idiots whilst working as a police officer to realise that being one myself would not be cool.

The nurses told us that I would be moved back to the ward that afternoon as I was now stable and awake, but first they needed me to get out of bed and stand up. This was apparently going to help with my recovery. I got to learn over the next few weeks just how important walking and movement was going to be for my physical recovery, but at that moment it felt like a crazy thing to be doing so soon after my operation.

They gave me a couple of hours to contemplate it before two of them suddenly loomed out of nowhere to help me perform a medical miracle. They said they needed me to demonstrate that I could get out of bed, albeit with assistance, before I could go to the ward.

There was a whirr as my bed lowered and another as my back was raised into a near sitting position. My heart was beating out of my chest and I was sweating as I swung my legs to the edge of the bed. The nurses took me under each arm as I tried to raise myself to a sitting position, and a cacophony of painful sensations erupted from my abdomen as I tried to raise myself up to a sitting position. It felt like my guts were going to spill out on to the floor in front of me.

I gritted my teeth and used my elbows to raise myself into a sit with the assistance of the nurses; I had absolutely no strength in my abdomen at all. I'm not sure what I expected having just been sliced in two, but the void of sensation and lack of strength across my middle was alarming. Looking down, I could see that my guts were clearly still inside me, so we carried on.

I shuffled on my bum to the edge of the bed, swung my legs down and planted my stockinged feet on the floor. This wasn't the moment to linger or be timid; it was too painful to be hanging about so I went straight into the stand. With a grunt I pushed myself up by my arms and simultaneously straightened my legs. The effort was huge, I couldn't believe how weak I felt. It was as if I'd been lying down for a month. My thighs were shaking uncontrollably underneath my gown but there I was standing up, albeit stooped over like a 90-year-old man. I couldn't straighten my back because it felt like there was an industrial elastic band from my neck to my groin pulling me tightly down into a curve. I tried to stretch it out but the pains came on very strongly, so I remained bent over looking at the floor.

Despite all this drama, the nurses seemed very pleased with my efforts and after a few seconds, which felt like minutes, they started to lower me back on to the bed and swung my legs up for me. As I slumped back, my chest was heaving and I could feel my back was cold with sweat against the mattress. I was completely physically exhausted. It took a few moments for the sharp stabbing pains to subside and as they did so I slipped into a deep morphine-induced sleep.

I rested like that in a more upright position for the rest of the afternoon before the porters arrived to take me back to the ward. I was unhooked from all the life support equipment and waved goodbye to the nurses as I was wheeled away in my bed with my bag-stand dragging along next to me and Maria scuttling along closely behind.

On the ward I was wheeled into the twin-intensive observation room and was backed up smoothly into my parking space. The nurses all cheerfully introduced themselves as I was hooked up to the monitoring equipment. There was a chap asleep in the bed opposite me who appeared to have as many tubes sticking out from under his bedclothes as I did. He was sound asleep despite the constant high-pitched beeping coming from a drip stand right next to his ear.

I was shown a small hand-held controller with a green button on it. This was my other new best friend: the morphine pump. It would allow me to self-administer set doses over set periods of time. I think it worked once every eight minutes or so and when it was ready to use the green light flickered back on.

I was constantly encouraged to use that little button by the nurses every time they came into the room, the theory being that if I lay there being a martyr to the pain it wouldn't help me relax and get better. A quick press of the button demonstrated that theory very well as I drifted away into a sweet morphine-induced haze for a few minutes. I spent a long time that day staring at that bloody button waiting for the green light to give me my next little fix.

I lay back and considered the shape I was in. It was 21 November 2014 and this was day zero for sure. I felt like a lump of meat and physically I was completely ruined. I still didn't know what other follow-up treatments I would need, but I told myself that I would get a little better every day until 13 September 2015 when I would be on that Ironman start line. In the meantime, I'll just lie back and have one more little press on my button.

Chemo Haze, All in My Brain

MY FIRST full day on the ward was a bit of a blur. I spent a lot of time drifting in and out of sleep. The pains in my abdomen were sloshing over me in sickly waves – if I lay very still I could ride them out until they subsided into the background. I felt like I was pushing my morphine button like mad but it didn't seem to be achieving very much in the way of relief. I was beginning to feel thoroughly miserable and had to work very hard not to break my rules about becoming an arse. I complained about the pain to the nurses and when they looked at my pump usage it turned out that I was only using about four doses an hour. Apparently I could have had up to twelve, so no wonder I was struggling. It wasn't my job at that very moment to help cut the National Health Service deficit so I started pressing the button with a bit more enthusiasm and it made a big difference.

I also had an opportunity to chat with the guy opposite me. His name was Rob and his operation had been a few days before mine. Our diagnosis stories were remarkably similar and at a similar age, with a similarly stupid sense of humour, we struck up a friendship straight away. His operation had been more invasive than mine by the sounds of it, but his prognosis seemed pretty good. His wife was staying in the same apartment on the hospital grounds as Maria, so they also had the chance to chat and unwind over several bottles of red wine of an evening.

That first afternoon I was due my first post-operative dose of chemotherapy. It would be administered directly into my abdominal cavity via the tubes inserted during my operation. It was a bit of a shock to see the nurses when they appeared with it – they looked like they were about to operate on a chimpanzee in one of those disease outbreak B-movies. They both had full-length bibs on with face masks and elbow-length rubber gloves. Bloody hell, if they were that worried about splashing it on to themselves what on earth was it going to do to my insides?

The chemo itself was dark brown and looked like black tea in a big clear plastic bag. It was hung on a hook above me and joined to a port attached to one of my drains. The port was then slowly opened and gravity was left to do the rest of the work. I watched the fluid come slowly down the tube and disappear into me. It took about an hour for the bag to be emptied and when it was done it felt like my stomach was pumped up like a beach ball with all that fluid inside me. It was a very uncomfortable feeling and within a few minutes I could feel a distant stinging sensation deep within. I pressed my button and lay back to let the treacly sensation of the morphine do its work.

I was feeling a bit groggy and my bloods had indicated that my oxygen levels were getting low, so I was given a mask to wear. It was one of those tubey types which wrap around your ears with two little nubs sticking up your nostrils to blow a cool trickle of oxygen directly into your nose. The cool air felt and smelt good and as I inhaled deeply I could instantly feel my head clearing a little.

I decided that I would move from the bed to the chair for a bit that evening and with Maria helping and a nurse in attendance, I was raised up to a sitting position on the bed and then shuffled slowly to the edge. My biggest problem was trying not to get tangled up in all my trailing tubes and pipes. We had to lift some over the bed, some had to be hooked over my little bag stand and the rest held up to stop them painfully pulling at the skin they were stitched into. I planted my feet on the floor and swung my backside straight around into the chair, but by the time I had rearranged my trailing tubes I was exhausted and was ready for another nap.

It was warm and clammy in the hospital and the morphine I was marinating in was now starting to make me itch and sweat badly. I was running with it; my brow was constantly beading up and sweat would drip from my nose like I was sitting in a sauna. My bed sheets were so drenched I needed them changed twice a day. I was lying and sitting on these big nappy-like pads to stop bed sores but these were also soaked through within minutes. I was lucky enough to have a fancy Dyson fan next to my bed and I tried to keep it blowing cool air over my itchy head at all times.

I was still pretty much nil by mouth, but I was given a carton of apple juice to sip, and the explosion of flavour on my tongue was incredible. It doesn't take long for you to appreciate flavours when you've had nothing but water for five days. To top everything else, I was now three days into a massive caffeine withdrawal and as a result my temples were pounding. I figured that it was a grotty addiction anyway and a bit of enforced cold turkey would sort me out. Maybe I'd go caffeine-free when I got out. Yep, like that worked out for more than a fortnight. I am still a confirmed caffeine freak who can't go more than four hours without getting a headache and the shakes.

Shuffling back into bed after an hour in my chair, I glanced down and to my horror saw what was the undeniable smear of a skid mark on the absorbent pad I had been sitting on. Being a self-confessed clean freak, it was crushingly embarrassing. I was completely helpless – it was now too far out of my reach for me to retrieve and hide without getting out of bed again and I wasn't going to be risking that, so I just had to sit there in mortified silence waiting for a nurse to appear. One duly strolled over and without a second glance folded it up and took it away. Not a word was said but I was left squirming uncomfortably around in bed wondering just how shitty my sweaty arse was and whether I'd be soiling any more bedding. I was completely helpless to do anything about it. No doubt I'd be getting a bed bath soon but would I have enough strength to wipe my own backside with a wet wipe or would I have to roll over for the nurse to do it? Bloody hell, what had become of me. My dignity was currently well and truly left at the door.

It's hard to describe just how bad the chemotherapy made me feel for those next few days. The doses were applied daily, with each dose lasting about 22 hours, the remaining two hours of the day allowed for the drainage of the previous dose and the administering of the next.

While the chemo was doing its thing, I can say without any shadow of a doubt that I have never felt so unwell or bereft of life. I would sit in the chair or lie in my bed blankly staring at the walls or ceiling. I slipped in and out of an exhausted, restless sleep during the day and then lay awake during some of the longest, loneliest nights I've ever had to endure.

My brain was fried by the chemicals. I couldn't concentrate for long enough to even listen to music or read a magazine; the treatment truly scoured my body from the inside out. I felt like my soul had been chased out and was hiding nearby watching and waiting to see if the empty husk of my broken body would survive long enough for it to consider coming back in.

The treatment was so poisonous, I could feel myself come back to life as the chemo drained away only to slip back into another sickly malaise as the next dose slowly dripped back in. Those days were long but I gritted my teeth and got through them. I was due to have four doses so I knew that it would all eventually be over and it was that thought that kept me going.

My parents were still visiting each day and Maria was with me most of the time but I just didn't have the energy to concentrate on conversation or answer the same old questions about how I was feeling, surely it was obvious wasn't it? I was feeling like shit and I was enduring a painful treatment which hopefully was going to save my life, what more did people want to know? The constant 'how are you feeling?', the questioning and the fussing attention irritated me so much that at times I just pretended to be asleep so I could be left alone. I was due a visit from Luigi but Maria had to put him off for a few days as I said I just wasn't up to it. I was busy breaking all my rules about being an arsehole.

By the third day I was feeling really low, but I knew that I had only one more day to go, so I just had to knuckle down and get it done. I still hadn't eaten anything and had only sipped on some water, so I was on a drip for hydration and my TPN was mainlining through my ribs all the sustenance I needed to survive, but despite it I was still feeling incredibly weak. I was told that the body can use up to 4,000 calories a day recovering from a serious operation. I had become a 24-hour-a-day calorie-burning furnace which was now well in deficit.

During the consultant's rounds on the fourth morning, Mr Mohamed explained that my blood results were showing that I had developed very low phosphate levels as a result of the chemotherapy. He had decided to withdraw the fourth and final round of treatment because of this. I protested, saying that I was prepared to go another 24 hours for the sake of my treatment, as I figured what was another day if it improved my chances for the rest of my life. Mr Mohamed was quite clear though and said that they were there to make me better, not finish me off. He convinced me when he said he was happy that the doses I had already endured were enough to give me the best chances possible, and as everything had gone so well so far he wasn't prepared to take any unnecessary risks with my health.

I had been warned by the nurses that morphine-induced hallucinations were a possible side effect to the high doses I had been receiving, and earlier that day I had been treated to my first, and, fortunately, only one. I was sat with Maria between chemotherapy doses and was having a brighter moment when I suddenly noticed all the curtains around the room were swaying from side to side. Not only were they swaying but they were pulsing up and down and moving as if they were breathing in and out. I told Maria what I was seeing and she confirmed that it was nothing that she could see. I clamped my eyes shut for a few moments but when I opened them again they were all still moving and this time the floor and the ceiling had joined in. We both properly laughed for the first time in ages as I stared around the room in wide-eyed wonder at the show the morphine was putting on for me. At least my pump appeared to be working at last, but I was subjected to a bouncy castle hospital for about two hours until it suddenly stopped just as quickly as it had started.

I was now being given strong paracetamol injections through a port in my cannula several times a day to supplement my morphine and I was surprised just how much relief I got in the hour or so following them. When I took paracetamol at home I always wondered if it really did anything, but here the effect was marked and the pain relief was very noticeable. I started using my pump less and held out for the injections.

As Rob was a couple of days ahead of me, the physiotherapists came for him and he had to do the first of many walks up and down the corridor. I watched him shuffle off out of the door being held up by each elbow and I laughed as he grunted and groaned his way down the corridor. The nurses told me not to laugh too loudly as I would be joining him in a couple of days. I said that we would therefore compete in the inaugural Cancer Ward Olympics to keep things interesting. Rob obliged and set the time to beat of about ten minutes for the first event, the assisted 50-yard shuffle.

The next day it was at last time for my first bed bath. I was starting to get a bit smelly and my hair was stuck to my head in a greasy mess so I was very grateful for the opportunity to freshen up. Maria was around and between the two of us and the nurse I managed to get a decent wash done whilst retaining a crumb of dignity. I only managed to make my eyes water the once when I tweaked on my catheter tube as I shuffled about on the bed.

It was also time to take the dressing off my wound to give it some air, and it was my first opportunity to take a proper look at the damage, which was quite impressive. I had 38 metal staples going in a line from my ribcage right down to my pubic bone. The wound itself was pinched together between them. My belly button was gone and the skin was visibly stretched across the space where it used to be. My whole belly was puffed up and swollen like an overstuffed sausage – it was numb to the touch with some evident nerve damage. What struck me most was the smell – there was the unmistakably sweet smell of rotting flesh when the dressing came off. Looking at the edges of the wound, it was yellow and damp, but I certainly wasn't expecting to find myself smelling like gone-off chicken.

After three of the very longest sweat-soaked miserable days of my life, my primary treatment was at last over and I was mightily relieved to be through it. As the last of the chemotherapy drained from me and the life started to drain back into me, my soul stopped hiding in the corner of the room and slipped back inside as the haze I had been existing in began to lift. At last it was time to start getting better.

A Dirty Protest and Drain Number Three

AFTER ANOTHER long night lying awake in what felt like non-stop sweaty morphine-soaked agony, I could finally sit up and get on with another daytime of sweaty morphine-soaked agony – it was seriously hard work. The night-times really dragged. The evening started to draw in at about 7:00 when the ward slowly ramped down for the night and the visitors and doctors started to thin out. The lights remained on until about 10:00, when they are dimmed in the rooms, but they remain on in full sun-like fluorescence in the corridors until much later. So if you are used to sleeping in the dark then you are out of luck.

Hospitals are also bloody noisy all day and all night. The constant beeping of alarms is the worst of it and it's usually caused by a bubble in a drip or something equally minor. The nurses seem to be able to tune it out and can let the beeping go on for hour after infuriating hour, until eventually someone will show up to press 'reset', only for it to start beeping again two minutes later. This goes on for 24 hours a day, so I would watch the 'bubble in the drip beep-stopping procedure' intently and eventually I got brave or frustrated enough to reach out, open up the machine and sort it out for myself. Along with the non-stop beeping, there are often random old people with dementia shuffling around the wards shouting angrily and refusing to go back to bed. Unlike some other well-known establishment, a good night's sleep is never assured in this hotel.

All you can do is lie there and stare at the ceiling or the inside of your eyelids and wait it out. I would lie in the gloom listening to Rob snoring and keep telling myself that it's just a waiting game and it will all be over at some point. This is what got me through those nights with nothing to do but wait for my morphine button to reset whilst waves of cramping rolled through my belly.

As another morning dawns, the hospital comes alive with the day staff rolling into work and the cleaners and medicine trolleys starting to clatter up and down the corridors. I got my breakfast of a child's size carton of apple juice and an orange jelly and started to feel a bit better, so after another refreshing bed bath and my daily round of blood samples given up to the vampires, I decided to mix it up again and sit back in the chair. I was starting to get adept at shuffling from the bed to the chair but it was still a fiendishly complicated procedure. Lift this tube over here, pass that tube under the other one, mind the catheter!

Once I was in the chair I instantly felt sick, my stomach was rock hard and I was swallowing back the spit gathering in my mouth. I grabbed a cardboard hat and held on tight waiting for the inevitable. Vomiting when you are being held together by a row of metal staples is disconcerting to say the least, and you definitely don't want to be popping a stitch.

When you have a bowel operation your whole digestive tract goes into shock – it's called an ileus. It wakes up slowly over a few days, but different parts can wake at different times which can cause complications. The stomach is continuously generating bile to digest food and this usually drains slowly into your bowels, but unfortunately your stomach doesn't talk to your bowels so when they go into ileus the bile has nowhere to go and builds up until your stomach is so full its only got one direction to release it and that's upwards.

Through experience I can tell you that about twice a day this process results in half a litre of bright green burning acid shooting out of your mouth and nostrils with alarming force. To avoid this unpleasantness the nurses will periodically put a big syringe into your nasogastric tube and suck out the entire contents of your stomach. The relief from this is instant and it became a bit of an obsession watching the green liquid filling the syringe.

It wasn't the best start to the day as I was shortly due to throw my hat into the ring for the Cancer Ward Olympics. The physiotherapists came to get me mid-morning and took me for my first stroll. With one on each side, they helped me stand up and together we shuffled out of the ward into the corridor for the first time. I was encouraged to stand as straight as I could but my incision was still pulling me tightly down into a stoop. I shuffled my way to the end of the corridor and back again in a new games record of about eight minutes and loudly declared myself the new record holder as I returned. Rob was unimpressed and said that he would be ready to smash that time out of the park in the morning. Maria watched me stagger off and took a photograph of me in the corridor as I shuffled along.

When I returned, exhausted and sore, to my chair, I looked at the picture and it became clear just how much work I had ahead of me if I was ever going to make it to the start line of that Ironman in ten months' time, let alone have any hope of completing it. I was told that the best thing I could do to help my recovery was move, and a daily walk of even a few metres was going to help enormously to get the scar tissue mobile. I told the physiotherapists of my Ironman intentions and they just stared at me blankly. They didn't really comprehend what an Ironman was and when I explained it their expressions still didn't change much. I took that as encouragement – at least they didn't laugh out loud or worse, tell me off.

After a bit of a sponge down I decided to go back to bed and get some sleep, as even the act of having a quick wash was completely exhausting. As I lay in bed I could see that the nurses had come to change Rob's dressings. The incision from his operation wasn't healing well and he needed to have his dressings changed daily, which was a very uncomfortable experience for him. We would often laugh at each other's misfortune and I sat up in bed and guffawed loudly as he groaned and cursed from behind the curtain on the other side of the room.

I was laughing and grimacing at the same time because the jiggling was really quite painful but it felt good to be in high spirits despite everything. Rob told me to bugger off and as I laughed I felt a gurgling inside me and let out a little fart. It was more of a grumble than a fart to be honest, but it took me by surprise and I instantly stopped laughing as I felt an unmistakable wetness between my butt cheeks. I called out to the nurses that I thought I may have had a little accident and it was Rob's turn to laugh. One of them called out from behind the curtain saying not to worry and they would come and have a look when they were done there.

As I shuffled uncomfortably from side to side in the bed, there was another unmistakable louder growl and burble from deep inside me and another more audible fart rumbled up from under the sheets. This was followed by an overwhelming wetness across the backs of my legs. I lifted the sheets and gingerly took a look. 'Yep, I've definitely had an accident.'

I was told to sit tight until the nurses could get to me. I didn't have the strength to lift myself out of the bed without making a right old mess so just had to lie back as the smell started to waft around the ward. The nurses went off and came back dressed in long gloves and plastic bibs. They were armed with a mountain of wet wipes, a hazardous waste bag and a big tub of soapy water. They seemed completely unfazed by the devastating scenes that they were being confronted with and seemed absolutely delighted that I had at least done some business. I, on the other hand, was completely and utterly mortified.

The curtains were drawn around us and by the time I had slid and wrestled my way to the edge of the bed for a second time that day, I was in a right old state. It looked like I'd been engaging in some sort of dirty protest by the time I managed to stand up next to the bed with the help of the two young nurses. I stood naked from the waist down, legs shaking like a frightened dog, whilst clinging to my drip stand for dear life as the nursing assistants wiped down my backside and testicles with tissues. My humiliation was complete; I stood and stoically submitted myself to the clean-up praying for it to be over quickly.

If the whole scenario could have got any worse, it was just about to. I heard my father outside in the corridor laughing with the nurses.

'Where's that boy of mine then, is he behind here, what's going on?' He was right behind the curtain by that point.

'STOP! Don't come in here! Fuck off and get a coffee or something. I'm a bit busy at the moment.'

The last thing I needed was him bowling in with his undoubtedly embarrassing and inappropriate banter.

As the nurses finished up, one of them said, 'Let me get that thing out for you now.' I had no idea what she was talking about as she reached behind me and tugged what looked like half of a toilet roll tube out from my backside. I blinked tightly and winced, what the hell is that? I didn't even know it was in there. She explained that it was to help me go without straining; well, it had certainly done that.

Once operation 'clean-up' was finished and my bed was remade, I could get back in and try to relax for a bit, although I would be more guarded before relaxing that much from now on, that was for sure. I ensured that I was well stocked up on absorbent pads to sit on for the next couple of days.

The rest of that day was spent in less dramatic fashion dozing and dosing myself, and as I lay back trying to read more than a page of my book without losing concentration, a nurse came through and told me that they would start to remove the drains from my abdomen the next day. I remembered how uncomfortable it was when the drain in my appendix was removed. This was a job for the nurse on the ward with no extra anaesthetic, they just cut the stitches holding the drain in place and slid it out with a firm tug. I had five of them this time though, not just the one, so that would be something else to think about whilst I lay awake during the night.

Maria was with me the next day when the nurse came to start the tube removal procedure. After the doctor's ward rounds it was decided that as the bile being pumped out through my nose was subsiding, they would also remove my NG tube, and as I was going to be more mobile after the drain removals they would also take out my catheter. That felt like real progress at last – I could begin to shed some of the tubes which were restricting my movement so much and maybe even lie on my side to get some sleep.

The catheter was removed in a single swift toe-curling yank and, in a similar no-nonsense manner, my nasogastric tube was whipped out with one long retching cough and the relief to be free of them both was instant. I was then given five minutes to press my morphine pump in preparation for the drain removals and we were ready to go.

I lay on the bed and held Maria's hand tightly as the stitches from around the first drain were snipped away. The nurse asked me if I was ready and I held my breath apprehensively as with the flourish of a magician pulling on a string of flags, the first drain was pulled out. The sensation was uncomfortable but not particularly painful; I could feel the tube uncurling from around my bowels as it slid out. It felt like a worm or snake was sliding around inside me. The second drain came out just as easily and I began to relax a little. It wasn't comfortable but it wasn't half as bad as I was expecting.

By the time the third drain was unstitched we all knew the drill and as she gave me the signal that she was going to pull I took another deep breath and exhaled, trying to relax through it. As soon as she started to pull, an instant agonising pain shot through my abdomen from deep inside my groin. It was so sharp and intense that I screamed out loudly. I have never screamed like that in my whole life and the volume and suddenness of it shocked everyone in the room. The nurse stopped pulling at once, as it was clear that this tube was stuck and wasn't in a hurry to slide anywhere.

I squeezed Maria's hand hard and could see that she was wide-eyed in shock and had turned as white as a sheet. I laughed nervously and tried to relax. My heart was galloping and I was breathing hard as the nurse prepared to give it another go. I breathed deeply through my nostrils and nodded that I was ready as she pulled again. Another wave of agony washed over me and I grunted from between my clenched teeth. I felt like one of my testicles was being pulled up inside me and waves of pain were radiating out from deep inside my groin, but the tube had barely moved a centimetre. Surely this wasn't right, I said to the nurse, and she told us that sometimes they can get a bit stuck but this felt like it had been stitched in.

Maria said that she felt faint and in the next instant she slid off of her chair and was lying under the bed staring up at the hydraulics; you're supposed to be supporting me, I thought.

While the nurse got Maria a glass of water and sorted her out, I took the opportunity to have a good press on my morphine pump and tried to relax. As the morphine kicked in, the pain subsided and Maria decided she would be better off waiting in the corridor as we decided to give it one more go.

'Ready?'

'Yes, do it.'

I felt a tearing sensation deep inside my groin and nearly passed out – the tube had moved a grand total of about two centimetres. I was physically shattered and I think the nurse was surprised by the difficulty and wasn't sure how to proceed. We agreed to stop and come back to it in the morning. I pressed my morphine button several times before the pain subsided enough for me to fall into a fitful, exhausted sleep for a few hours. That, without doubt, was the most painful thing I had ever experienced in my life and it wasn't even over yet.

I had another sleepless night worrying about it before the morning came and it was time to try again. Maria decided it was best if she was elsewhere this time and went for a coffee – she didn't want to end up being the patient again.

It was a different nurse this time but she was aware of the drama that had gone on the day before so between us we devised a strategy: I would dose up on the morphine between pulls and hopefully it was dislodged sufficiently to come out easier today. It wasn't to be. The first pull made me shout out again, nothing had changed and it was still stubbornly lodged in place. Pain was starbursting across my abdomen from the ripping sensations deep inside me and the tube had moved all of another centimetre. I re-dosed and tried to relax but my heart was racing and the adrenaline was pumping. I gripped on to the side of the bed with both hands as she pulled again and this time I physically saw the stars. It felt like someone had stabbed me in the balls with a red hot knife and I thought I was going to be sick.

As we waited for another dose of morphine to become available, I shakily asked if anything else could be done. She told me that it just needed to come out, if she called a consultant he would be annoyed and would simply pull on it harder than she was doing. I was starting to get really worried now because what was happening didn't feel like normal procedure to me. It felt like it was starting to do some real damage inside me – surely there was something a bit more scientific to it? If this was how it was, though, then there was nothing else for it, so we agreed to give it another go.

I told her this time to pull it hard and not stop till the bloody thing was out.

She pulled and I grunted again through my gritted teeth. I felt it dislodge and as it started to slide she physically stumbled back as it finally freed itself. I shouted out loudly in relief, 'It's out! It's fucking well out! Well done!' I slumped back on the bed relieved and exhausted.

I looked down at the two remaining drains and my heart sank, please don't make me go through all that again. I took a deep breath and, despite my terror, the two remaining drains slid out with relative ease, much to everyone's relief. Rob and his wife had been sitting quietly on the other side of the room with white faces witnessing the drama and congratulated me on getting it done. They looked as shocked as everybody else by what had just occurred.

With the tubes out and my body full of morphine, I found that I could roll on to my side a little and into a more natural sleeping position. So, propped up by my pillows for the first time since the operation, I fell into a deep sleep. I woke up refreshed just in time for lights out.

Fifty Shades of Green

AFTER ANOTHER long night lying on damp sheets, I was starting to get a bit ripe again. I was beginning to smell like one of the zombies in my comics and it wasn't a pleasant prospect for anyone who had to get near me, so I was delighted when the nurses told me I could take a proper shower.

I was much more mobile now without all of the tubes sticking out of me but I still had to be careful because of my epidural and my PIC line which were attached to some very delicate parts of my body and still very much needed. I was weak on my feet and was struggling to stand upright so I definitely needed assistance to successfully take a shower, and fortunately Maria was around to help me out so I didn't have to bare my backside to another nurse.

After a breakfast consisting of another child-sized apple juice, it was time to hit the showers. Maria helped me to the cubicle and I shuffled around and sat down heavily on to the plastic chair that had been positioned behind the curtain for me. I slipped off my gown and sat naked and shivering waiting to be hosed down. Maria held the shower hose above my head and the warm water that started to run over me felt wonderful. I relaxed as Maria washed my hair, closing my eyes and enjoyed the feeling of the water on my skin.

Out of the cubicle and dressed in a fresh gown, I felt good. The warmth of the water had loosened my muscles and I took a moment to lean back and stretch out my abdomen. It still felt as if there was an elastic band pulling me down but I managed to half straighten up and relieve some of the tension in my back and shoulders, which clicked alarmingly. I lifted my chin and looked around at the walls instead of the lino floor I was more accustomed to seeing as I waddled about.

Sat back in my chair, my scar was really stinging from the soap but I was still feeling good. I could sense my body was already beginning to heal and it was very encouraging. A couple of presses on the morphine pump dulled the pain and I sat back and found that I had the concentration to read a magazine for the first time. That honeymoon period didn't last long though and within the hour the morphine itches were back with a vengeance and drips of sweat were once again running off my nose and on to the magazine I was reading.

Despite the progress I felt I was making, I was brought firmly back down to earth with a bump later that day when I went down for my first proper physiotherapy session. In the mini gym at the end of the corridor I was subjected to what can only be described as the beasting from hell. My personalised full-body workout consisted of:

Five stand up and sit downs from a chair, ten step up and step downs from a small step, ten bicep curls with a one-kilogram dumbbell, followed by ten lateral arm raises using the same weight. I was then finished off with two minutes of seated cycling on a little pedal machine with no resistance. Cross fitters eat your heart out!

At the end of all that I was a broken man and needed to be taken back to my bed in a wheelchair. I spent the rest of the afternoon fast asleep.

Lunchtime that day I was asked what I fancied to eat and was treated to a tiny bowl of Heinz tomato soup, which was apparently a special order from the kitchen. I was allowed the luxury of deviating from the fixed menu by virtue of being a patient on one of the specialist wards. Who needed a private hospital with service like this? It was fantastic but the thimble it was served in did leave me feeling a little bit short-changed. I noticed for the first time in a long time a growling in my stomach and realised I was starting to get a bit hungry. I hadn't had that sensation since before my operation and it was a good indication that my bowels were starting to reverse direction and flow downward again.

I was now starting to eat solids, so my consultants decided to remove my PIC line, meaning I was free from yet another of my tubes. I was worried about this one being removed as it was sticking straight out from between my ribs in the top of my chest. But I needn't have worried as after a good hit of morphine it slid out so easily I didn't even feel it. This was good news but meant that I would have to rely solely on my stitched-up bowels for sustenance from now on.

That evening I ate my first proper meal of a small piece of indeterminable white fish and some mashed potatoes. It was so good to feel the texture of real food in my mouth and to chew and taste something properly. Although the portion was small I struggled to eat it and after just a few mouthfuls I was feeling like I was forcing it down. I only managed one more small spoonful of mash before giving up. I've always had a good appetite but I didn't want to push it too hard too soon.

What followed was easily the worst night of my entire stay in hospital, as it appeared that I had overdone it at dinner after all. Painful cramps were rolling around inside me and I had to draw my legs up to my chest to get some relief. The morphine wasn't even touching them, so in the middle of the night the on-call doctor had to come to the ward to prescribe me an extra dose of paracetamol to help take the edge off.

It felt like I had a rock-hard football inside me and I was swallowing back the saliva all night until at four in the morning the inevitable happened. I was dozing at the time and being taken totally by surprise by the speed of its arrival, I only just managed to grab the cardboard bowl I'd strategically placed by my bed earlier in the evening. Ridiculously loud retching rolled around the sleeping ward as a powerful jet of bright green fluid flew out of my nose and mouth. I thrust the bowl under my chin as a second squirt filled it right to the brim. I managed to splutter out to the nurse for another bowl and she rushed in just in time to catch the third projectile as it splashed over both our hands.

The relief was instant but by nine that morning I knew I was once again on the verge of another explosion. The green acid was back flying and this time it was moving with such force it hit the bottom of the cardboard bowl and bounced back out all over my bed sheets. Through the tears, I squinted and tried to angle the bowl in the right direction to catch the second salvo but it flew straight over the top and landed between my legs.

After a shower and shave to clear my head, I felt much better and was ready to discuss my progress with Mr Mohamed. He said it was likely my bowels were back in ileus as a reaction to the food and I would need to rest them a little longer to allow them time to recover. He assured me that this was often the case and was all perfectly normal. As he was leaving the room I put on another show for his benefit and filled another two bowls right to the brim. As he left Mr Mohamed joked that he didn't usually have that sort of effect on his patients.

My morphine pump just wasn't touching the cramping bowel pain, so that afternoon, in consultation with the doctor, we turned off the background dosage, which meant that I was now in sole control of my pain relief. Morphine can have a side effect of slowing the bowels and causing constipation so by reducing my dosages I could hopefully speed up my recovery.

Surprisingly, the only thing that was helping with the deep bowel pain was the paracetamol, so I took a rash decision to go cold turkey from the morphine. I tucked my button out of sight at the side of the bed and

I didn't press it again. The pain wasn't any less but the sweating and itching stopped pretty much straight away and my head felt a lot clearer. I was happy to take the discomfort in exchange for feeling more like my old self for the couple of hours between paracetamol doses. The downside was that if the medicine cart was late doing its rounds, I spent a lot of time getting increasingly irritable and uncomfortable waiting for my next fix, and the temptation to press the morphine button was massive.

Due to the ileus I was off the solids and back on the jelly. The concern now was that if I couldn't keep that down I wouldn't be getting any sustenance at all as my PIC line was now out. Every time I was sick the nurses had to measure it and it was averaging out at about 500 millilitres at a time, and I was barely sipping at my drinks so was now starting to dehydrate at an alarming rate.

That night the cycle of vomiting continued and I was becoming physically worn down by the effort of it. My staples and abs were screaming with every convulsion and my throat was burning from the bile. I was becoming increasingly more exhausted, so at around three in the morning the night nurses came to me and it was clear they needed to reinsert the nasal gastric tube. The last one was inserted when I was under anaesthetic and I hadn't yet had the pleasure of the procedure whilst awake, and the apologetic tone of the nurses told me it wasn't going to be very pleasant. It was a necessary evil though, as I was becoming far too weak to keep on vomiting at that intensity.

The tube itself looked far too thick to go up my nose when it was unravelled from its sterilised bag. Some

KY Jelly was applied to the end of it which made me chuckle and I was told to tilt my head back slightly and to continuously swallow as it went down. The nurse began to push it into my nostril and I sniffed as it hit the back of my nose and started to scratch as it prodded its way around. It got stuck after about three centimetres and no amount of painful pushing was making it go in. Apparently I have a kink in my left nostril which wouldn't let it pass through. I remembered that the previous tube was in the right side so we swapped nostrils and tried again. With a little more lubrication and some firm prodding, I was swallowing and gagging like a wide-eyed madman as the tube slid down into the back of my throat.

I had about ten seconds' grace before all the swallowing wiggled the tube and I started to retch as my gag reflex began to protest to its presence. I tried to relax but each time the tube moved, another wave of retching would start and I struggled for the next ten minutes in endless cycles of coughing and retching until the tube somehow nestled into a more comfortable position and I could catch my breath. Once again I was lying in bed covered in flecks of green sick.

That night I also went back on to a drip to get some much-needed fluids into me. I was so dehydrated the junior doctor and the senior nurse couldn't get a cannula to hit one of my deflated veins, and 30 painful minutes of pricking at both my elbows and forearms saw them give up and request the assistance of the on-call consultant. He was less than pleased to be taken away from whatever he was up to at silly o'clock in the morning to carry out such a minor procedure. He then proded around painfully for ten minutes himself, getting increasingly agitated as he couldn't find a vein either. I lay back quietly and tried not to make a fuss, and in the end he plunged it awkwardly into my wrist. It was a crappy position that stung every time I moved my hand and meant the tubes were constantly in my way every time I tried to pick something up, so in the afternoon I asked to have it moved once my veins were inflated enough to see again.

I felt like I was going backwards. I had just been released from all the trailing tubes and now I was back pushing a drip stand around everywhere I went. After such good progress this was a real setback and was really disappointing.

The nurses and all the doctors were convinced that it was just a matter of time before I was back on track, but it didn't feel like it. Although you don't really share them publicly, dark thoughts do creep into your head. What if it doesn't get any better, what then? The prospect of that was very frightening. I was just starting to adjust to the new me but this was always on the understanding that I would eventually be back to some sort of normality. If this was as good as it was going to get then I was in real trouble. I was feeling very weak now and in the mirror my cheeks were sunken and the face looking back at me was ashen and tired. I was visibly starting to waste away.

That night I kept the nurses on their toes by insisting on my stomach being aspirated every couple of hours and I was feeling a lot more comfortable as a result. I was certainly glad to see that green crap sucked up into a syringe instead of being in my lap.

Just a Little Prick Sir

EVEN THOUGH I appeared to be withering away, I was beginning to feel stronger as each day passed. The morphine was fading from my system and although I was still in a lot of pain it all felt very different. I now had a direct pain response to what I was doing and I could judge my body so much better without the fog of the drugs all over me.

I had been encouraged to get up and walk about as much as possible as it was the best way to help my intestines settle and keep my scar tissue from binding me up completely, and it also helped avoid any deep-vein thrombosis or blood clots which could develop from long periods of sitting about. So each morning and afternoon I would take a stroll up and down the ward, each time walking further and further. So far, in fact, that I was now getting tantalisingly close to the doors of the ward and planned my great escape for later in the day.

With the help of Maria, I stepped off the ward for the first time in two weeks and the plan was to walk down to one of the gardens for some fresh air. As I was back on a drip, I couldn't drag my stand and bag down the stairs so we had to take the lift to the ground floor, but this was still the furthest I had walked since the operation and it was seriously hard work. I was sore and tired and had to lean against the wall of the lift as we went down. I think the nurse who got in with us was worried I was going to have a funny turn before she could get out.

Fortunately the gardens were just a short walk from the lift and we were soon at the doors. I was wearing a hospital robe with my dressing gown over the top and shuffling along in my slippers. I looked every bit the hospital patient. I noticed people looking at me and I could tell that they were wondering what was up with me.

As soon as we got outside into the milky December sunlight, the cold air hit me like a slap around the face and it felt fantastic. I had been breathing in the warm shitty bowel ward air for two weeks solid and it felt like I had just stepped out into a ski resort; I gulped at the air like a goldfish. For the first time I thought how nice it would be to be out of the hospital and back home. It surprised me just how institutionalised I had already become in such a short amount of time.

My little bid for freedom couldn't last forever though, and we arrived back just in time for the medicine trolley to rattle its way on to the ward. In addition to all my pills, I had now started to be given a daily injection of blood-thinning medication. The nurses would either stick it in my thigh or in a pinch of skin in my stomach while I swallowed down my painkillers.

I was just about to present a shapely leg to the nurse when she surprised me by saying, 'Here you go, you can do it today,' and proceeded to pass me the packet with the syringe in.

I laughed. 'No thanks, you're alright, you carry on,' I replied worryingly.

She then looked at me with a much more serious face and said, 'Well, you need to get used to it, you will be doing it at home for yourself for the next month.'

This was the first I had heard of it but I could see she wasn't joking.

I took the packaging and she told me not to worry as she would talk me through it. I fumbled to open the plastic seal and took out the syringe. It was one of those all-in-one type affairs where you crack open the end to expose the needle, push it in and press down on the plunger. I bared a thigh and squeezed up a pinch of skin between my fingers. I could feel a bead of sweat quivering on my brow and my heart was pumping. I had to tell myself out loud to calm down, much to everyone's amusement.

I held the syringe shakily in my right hand and pointed the needle at the little bulge of skin I had pinched tightly between my fingers. I made a half-hearted jab for it and the needle stopped involuntarily a few millimetres away from the skin with a little bead of medicine jiggling on the end of it. I took a deep breath, licked my lips and tried again. It was like there was a physical barrier between me and the point of the needle as it hovered just above my leg and the little bead of medicine on the end of it dripped coldly on to me.

'Just relax,' came the not-very-useful words of encouragement from the nurse. I was beginning to feel like a bit of a wimp so it was time to get a grip of myself and get it done. I held my breath and slowly and deliberately pressed downwards and the needle slid under the skin. I gingerly pressed down on the plunger until it clicked and that was it, I had successfully injected myself for the first time in my life. 'That wasn't too bad in the end,' I winced. 'Jolly good, you can do it yourself from now on then,' said the nurse as she wheeled the trolley towards her next unsuspecting victim.

On that afternoon's shuffle around the ward I must have been feeling better as I managed to bend down and pick a mobile phone off the floor for a lady in one of the side rooms who was in danger of falling out of her bed while trying to reach for it, a feat of dexterity that even two days before would have defeated me. With each walk I could feel myself getting a little stronger but I got a bit carried away the next morning when I decided to walk to the shop at the front of the hospital to get myself a newspaper.

I compounded it by taking the stairs, which felt like a victory at the time until halfway back when I had to find a bench to sit on for 20 minutes to recover sufficiently to get myself to the lift and back into the safety of the ward.

The nurses were still aspirating an alarming amount of green bile from my nostrils, but as a direct result I wasn't feeling or being sick all the time. If I felt like I was filling up I just requested an extra suck which always seemed to do the trick.

The next morning I had my first cup of tea since I'd been admitted and although it was hospital tea and I had to swallow it past the tube in my throat, it still tasted bloody great. I was still on the drip for hydration and hadn't really eaten for two weeks, but I still had absolutely no appetite whatsoever and I could feel myself getting thinner by the day. The discussion was that if my ileus didn't settle soon I would need to go back on the TPN and a new PIC line would need to be inserted into my chest. I really didn't like the thought of that procedure, remembering the drain that had been inserted into my appendix, but I couldn't go much longer without any sustenance. I just had to hope that my aspirations started to reduce, and quickly.

Off the morphine I was feeling more like my old self all the time and even managed to get dressed by passing the IV line and bag through the sleeve of my t-shirt. I was still in a lot of pain and now very weak when I moved about, but the fact that I washed, dressed and sat in a chair all by myself felt like a great improvement over lying on a sweaty bed with my arse hanging out of the back of an ill-fitting hospital gown.

Late that afternoon I was wheeled back into a private room at the end of the ward. I was getting a visit from my sister that day and she had the shock of her life when she walked into the ward and saw an old man lying in my bed space. I think she genuinely thought I'd snuffed it during the night. With a wobbly lip she asked the nurse where her brother was and was directed to my private suite at the end of the ward where I was hiding. It was so good to have some peace and quiet, and that night, because I was feeling a lot better, the nurses let me push the door closed a bit, and shielded from the worst of the noise and light I slept soundly for a few hours.

It was now 3 December and I had been in hospital for 14 nights. I was due my histology results any day now, and with each passing consultant's round, the anxiety about the results was starting to build. The implications were crystal clear: if the cancer had spread to the lymph nodes it could mean that the cancer had spread from my body cavity to my organs. This would certainly mean follow-up chemotherapy of some kind and further complications. The grade of the cancer they removed would also give me an indication of the chances of a recurrence.

The implications for any training schedule were stark, I already had no idea how I was going to recover in time to start some serious training. If I needed regular chemotherapy there would be a very hefty knock-back. I dealt with the anxiety by thinking about the impact it would have on my training, which was much easier on the mind than thinking about the reality of the impact on my life expectancy or my chances for a healthy future.

Today, however, was going to be the day I got my results delivered during the consultant's rounds. As Mr Dayal said the words 'We've had your histology results returned,' my heart was in my mouth. Luckily he didn't make me wait with a dramatic reality-TV type pause and he followed up quickly with, 'But I'm pleased to say it's very good news.' I blew out my cheeks, sighed and sank back on to the bed as he went on to deliver the news.

All the lymph nodes that were removed from the bowel and surrounding area were tested and no spread of disease to them was detected. The three nodules of cancer that were removed from my abdomen were found to be of a medium grade, which effectively meant that, as they believed they had removed all the cancer, they thought the chances of a recurrence were relatively low. I would therefore not require further treatment other than an annual blood test and a scan to monitor my progress. I could see on his face how pleased he was to deliver the news. He had told me previously how happy he was with the outcome from the initial operation and he was now effectively giving me permission to go off and live my life. This was great news that I couldn't wait to share with Maria and then everybody else.

Once the doctors had moved on I was left alone in my room to digest the news. 'Thank fuck for that,' I said out loud to nobody in particular – the relief was immense. I wasn't completely in the clear but the news was as good as it could have been in the circumstances. Maybe I was going to live to be an old man after all. My thoughts then drifted to all the other patients on the ward. It was blindingly obvious that some were very sick indeed and not as lucky as I was, that was for sure.

Lucky seems like a strange word to use when you are talking about being diagnosed and treated for a dangerous and rare cancer, but for me it felt very appropriate. What hand did I play in my good outcome? Not a lot, and that went for every other person in that ward. There are so many variations and so many different factors involved and not many can be influenced by the patients themselves, so when I say I was lucky, I truly felt very lucky indeed.

My introspection was cut short by the senior nurse who came in to remove some of the staples which had been doing such a grand job of holding me together. The wound underneath them had been healing nicely and in the last couple of days it had even stopped smelling like a dead rat under the bedclothes. She produced a giant-sized office staple remover to do the job with and I pulled up my t-shirt and lay back as she got to work. The staples said goodbye with a click and a last little sting as they popped out one by one and clinked into the kidney bowl next to me on the bed.

Another milestone in my recovery was met but I still wasn't eating anything other than an orange jelly for breakfast. My bowels were stubbornly not waking up and with each aspiration of my tube, the green liquid kept on flowing until suddenly that evening it appeared that I was at last turning a corner.

I wasn't expecting anything different but as the nurse pulled on the syringe, strong suction held the plunger firmly in place. A couple more firm pulls put only about 100 millilitres into the syringe. This was really good news as suddenly it appeared that at long last my bowels were beginning to drain away my stomach contents. That evening for the first time I felt some painful twinges and gurgles inside me as my bowels gingerly plucked up the courage to restart the conveyor belt for a second, and hopefully last, time.

The nurse offered to take out my nose tube that evening but was surprised when I said I'd hang on to it for a bit longer. I didn't fancy a repeat of the last insertion and I had become somewhat attached to my trunk, so I opted to keep it in a bit longer to be on the safe side. As a compromise they removed the bag from the end of it and clamped it with a clip. This was a vast improvement as it wasn't swinging around and making me gag any more I was yet another degree better.

The next morning I woke up hungry for the first time which was a good sign, and when the breakfast trolley came around I treated myself to a small portion of Rice Crispies and a cup of tea. I managed about four mouthfuls before I felt full but restrained myself by remembering the consequences from the last time I over-ate by two bites. My stomach gurgled alarmingly for the rest of the morning but other than that I seemed to be keeping it down.

I even went to the toilet for the first time. It may have been just a drop of medicated rusty-coloured water, followed up with some bowl-rattling wind, but it was a great cause for celebration on the ward. I even had to leave it so that the nurse could inspect it. Who knew that there was an official guide for measuring the firmness of your stools? I was a solid seven on the Bristol Scale.

That afternoon I had the last of my staples taken out and lost the drip and the nose tube as I was now back drinking water again. I sat dressed and comfortable on my bed and realised how much I had improved in just a few short days. I was still walking like a 90-year-old man with a broken back, but within myself I felt so much stronger and more alert. I could even start to feel my abdominal muscles again. I pulled my t-shirt up and watched as I gently squeezed them, but instead of tightening evenly across my belly it was weird to see on one side of the scar the muscles tightening upwards and inwards while the other side did the exact opposite. There was some real damage down there, that was for sure.

Providing I ate something and didn't have any further reactions, the consultants were pleased to tell me that I could go home the next day. Free from all my tubes, that evening I rolled on to my side, and although it was quite painful to have my belly hanging down, I was at last back in my natural sleeping position and I slept the whole night like a log.

So after nearly three weeks in hospital I was at last going home. I showered, dressed and waited and then waited some more. I was fully expecting to be out by lunchtime, but it was already 11:30 and the consultants were late for their rounds.

I had some lunch and another cup of tea and the sign-off came around 1:00 in the afternoon with smiles and handshakes all round. I just had to wait for my medicine to come up from the pharmacy and I could go home. I found Rob in another side room and wished him all the best for the future. Despite everything that had happened to us over the last few weeks we had definitely made the most of it by keeping each other laughing and I was very grateful for his company. He was due to be discharged the next day and had spent a little longer in hospital than me due to some complications of his own. It also looked like he hadn't been lucky enough to dodge the follow-up chemotherapy like I had and would require further treatment. I often think of him and wonder how he is getting on now.

It was nearly 4:00 in the afternoon now and I was in danger of the pharmacy closing without getting my medication. I was very close to having to stay another night so several calls were made and we were told that we could collect my prescription on our way out as there had been a mix-up and they were about to close the pharmacy, so that was it, we were off. I walked along the ward for the last time, said goodbye to the nurses and presented them with a card and a box of chocolates to go with the piles of treats they seemed to have collected from every patient who had ever left the ward. How they weren't all 20 stone is beyond me.

Maria carried my bag to the car and I sat in the winter sun on a bench by the doors trying to enjoy some fresh air along with all the smokers. I watched patients and visitors coming and going and it already seemed surreal that I had just spent three weeks going through what they were all still going through.

It was another key moment in my life sat there in the sun – I had to walk the talk now to get this Ironman done. Physically I could not have been weaker or more damaged. I had a long way to go and the path ahead was certainly going to be a difficult and painful one, but this was the time to step up and own the rest of my life whatever it was going to look like. I had relied on others to get me better till this point and now it was my turn.

One thing I did know for sure was that I had changed; it was a subtle change but the old me was gone. The 'lazy, that will do' attitude of old was in the past. I had just shy of ten months to plan and execute the challenge of a lifetime, which under normal circumstances would have been a real feat to achieve. The old me would never have even considered it.

Sat on that bench I was at zero – the only way I could go from here was forwards and upwards and it was a very positive feeling.

I didn't feel angry that I had cancer, I didn't feel sad or resentful for the uncertainty I was facing. Fuck the cancer, it was now all about living, not worrying about biological changes inside me that I had no control over.

I was grateful for the reset button being pressed on my life, rolling through life was no longer acceptable. I had faced my mortality and now understood my life, in fact all life, better. I had an acceptance of death which I was previously blind to and in turn it meant that I had a better appreciation of what it meant to be living. I wasn't going to waste my life any longer by marking time or settling for second best. It still felt like an impossible dream to do an Ironman, but could it be possible if I put my mind and body to it? Why not?

After a few minutes Maria appeared with the car and swung it around into the patient pick-up area. As she helped me into the passenger seat, I don't think she realised she was about to drive away a new husband already bursting with possibilities. If I failed at this bloody Ironman it wouldn't be for a lack of trying, that was for sure.

Home Sweet Home

ARRIVING BACK at the house I slumped into my favourite leather armchair and looked around. It was good to be home. The drive back from the hospital had been a very uncomfortable one. I had to hold the seat belt out from my scar and the constant jolts and rattles coming through the suspension from the high-quality British roads made for a long and painful journey. I pressed my feet into the footwell and tried to lift my backside off the seat to relieve the lightning bolts shooting through me from the worst of the potholes. The stress of my time in hospital also appeared to have rendered Maria unable to drive and I gritted my teeth through a 40-minute kangaroo ride across every junction till we eventually pulled up on the driveway.

It's the subtle things that make you relax when you are back in the familiar surroundings of your own home. You don't notice it until you've been away for a good while but the feel of a chair or the carpet under your feet makes you feel instantly comfortable. The smell of your own home and being surrounded by your own possessions definitely gives you an enormous sense of well-being.

As I sat back and gently lifted my legs on to the pouffe, I realised just how bloody noisy and stuffy it was in hospital. Luigi had said to me that in his view hospitals were disease-infested shit pits and the quicker I was home the better. Maybe a bit harsh but sat back in my chair I could certainly understand the sentiment.

That night I was in bed exhausted by eight, but the silence was deafening and I couldn't get to sleep. It was my first night lying flat in bed as I was always at least a bit propped up in hospital. As I twisted and turned in bed I could feel my guts moving and sliding inside me and my scar stretching. I ended up with about three hours of fitful sleep sat bolt upright propped up on about six pillows. It certainly wasn't the good night's sleep I had been dreaming about for the last three weeks.

Back at home I naturally had to start managing my own food. I was still suffering from diarrhoea about twice a day and I had been told to start easy on a low fibre, low volume diet. Things like white bread and doughnuts were recommended to keep the fibre down but get the much needed calories into me. I weighed in at the hospital at 88 kilos but standing on the scales at home I was now just 79. In three weeks I had lost over nine kilos and my weight was still sliding south. A couple of kilograms I could put down to the offal they removed on the operating table, but the rest was all loss of fat and muscle mass. Looking in the mirror I

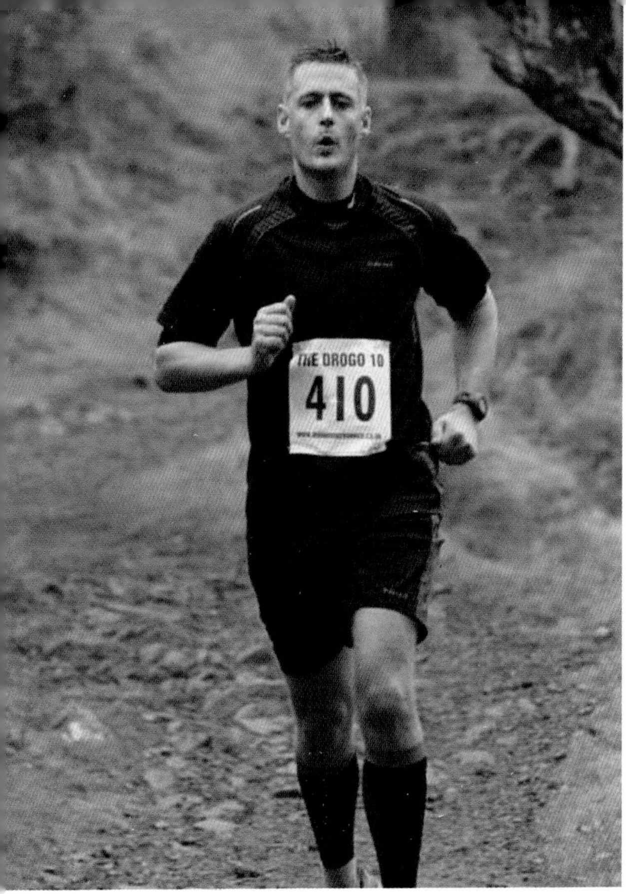

Chasing down the opposition at the Drogo Ten

Laying in an induced coma in intensive care after the Mother of all Surgery

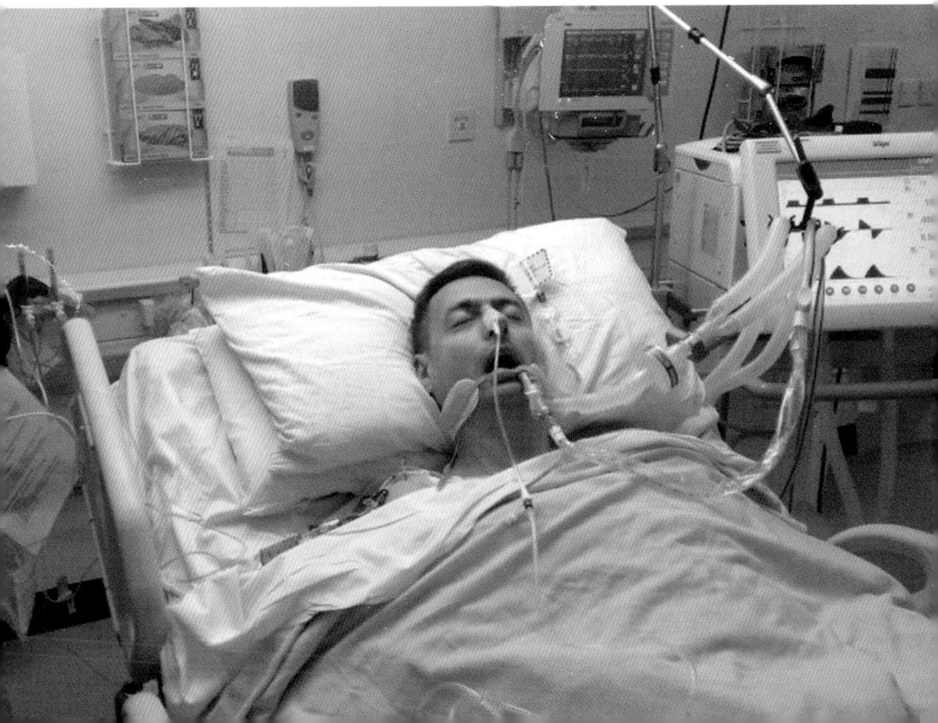

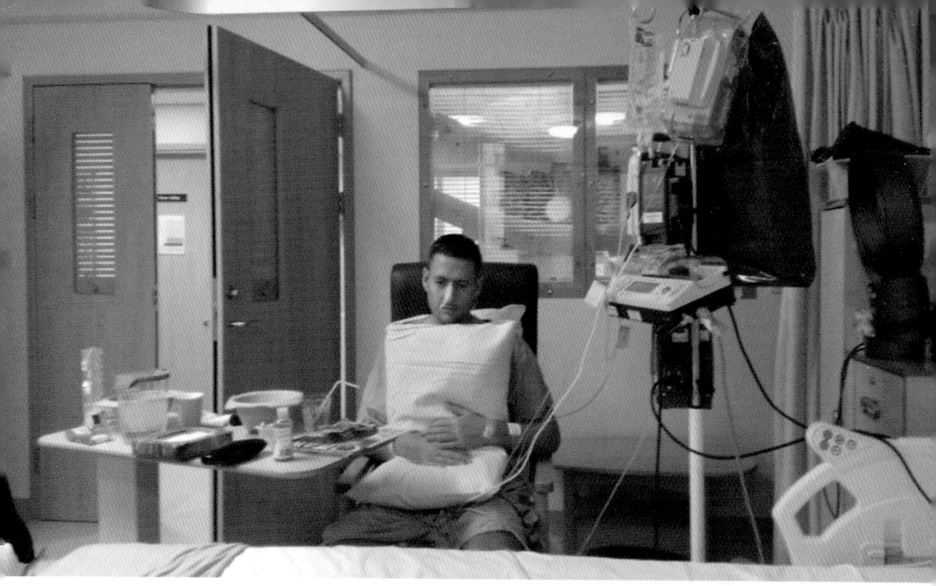

Getting through the day with a belly full of chemotherapy

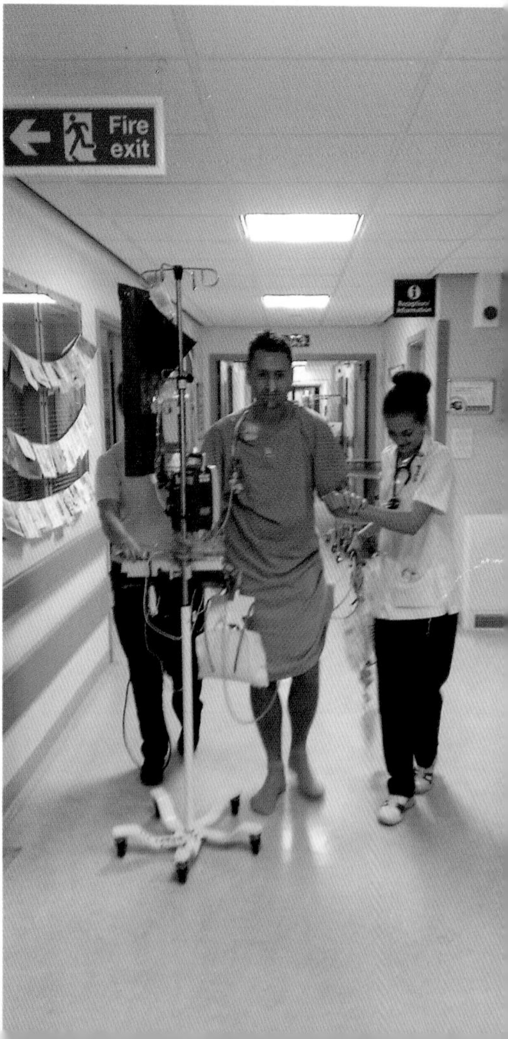

My debut 50 metre shuffle in the Cancer Ward Olympics

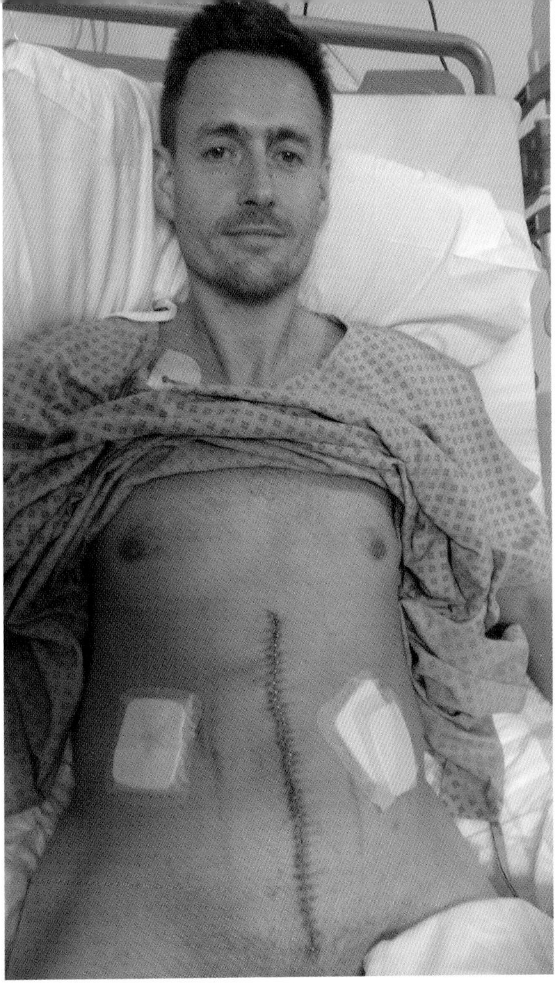

My operation scar in all its glory shortly after the removal of drain number three

First bike ride post-surgery on a very chilly January morning

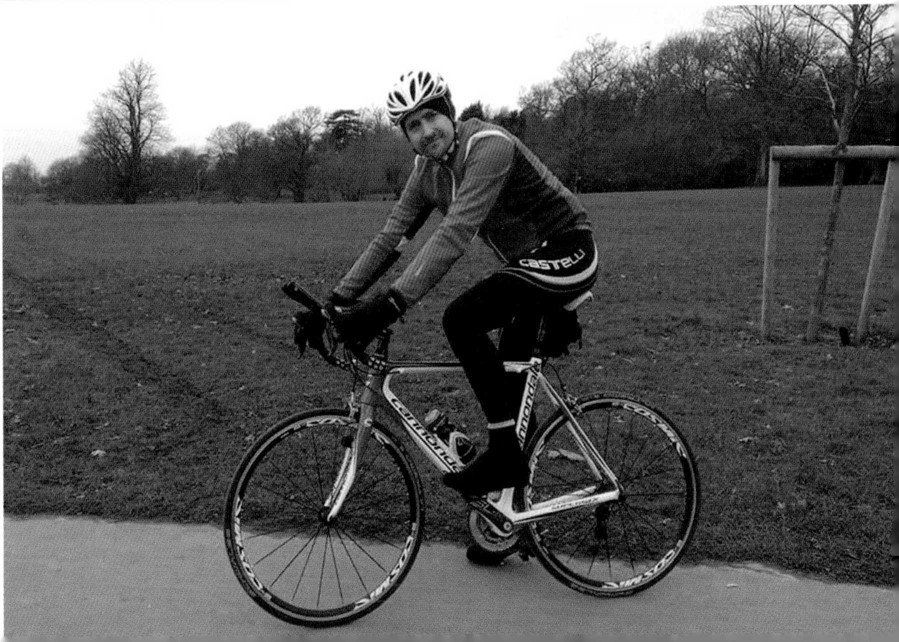

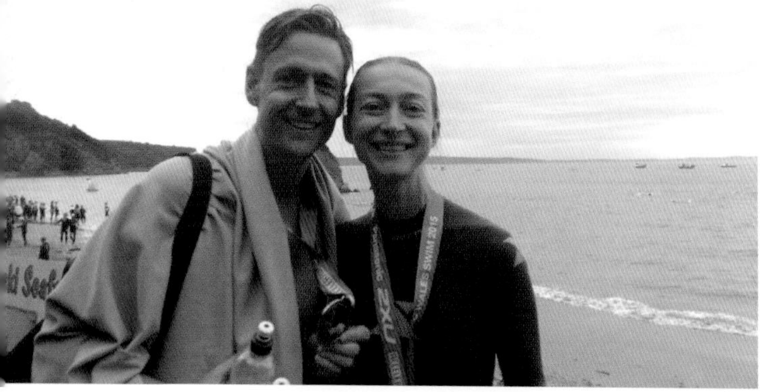

Chuffed to bits after our first competitive open water swim at the Long Course Weekend

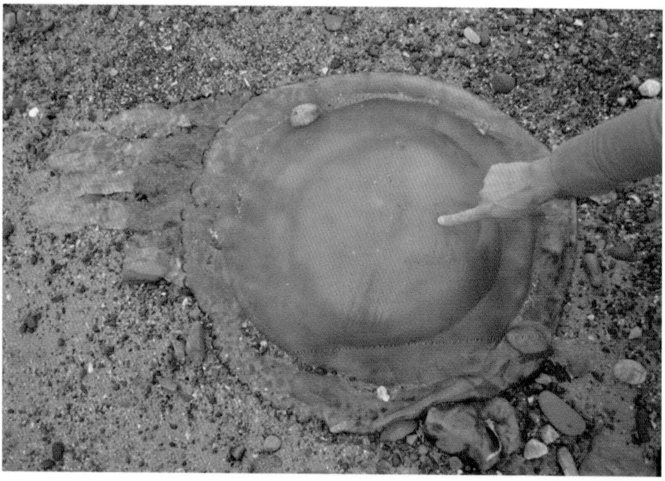

A killer jellyfish at Tenby North Beach

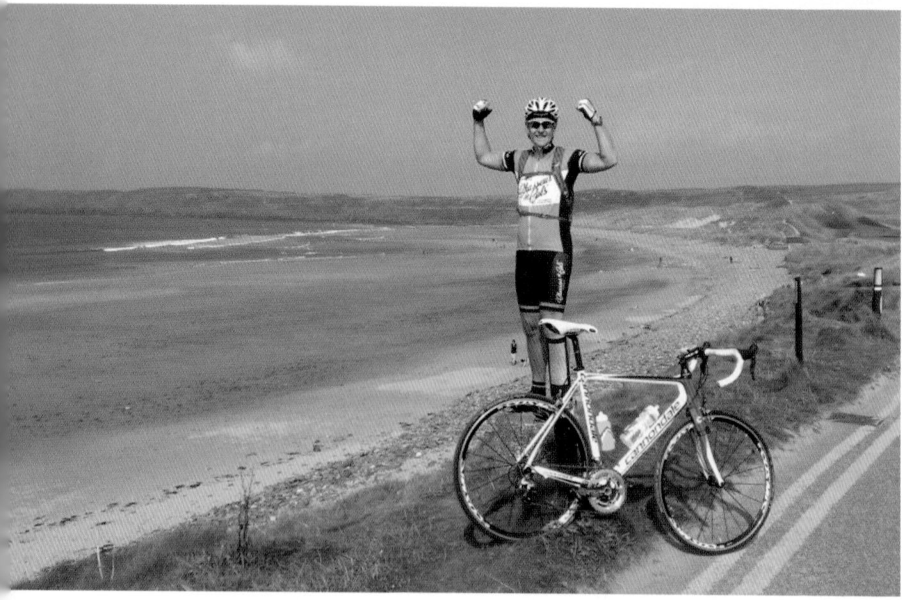

Feeling on top of the world on a recce ride to Freshwater West, Pembrokeshire

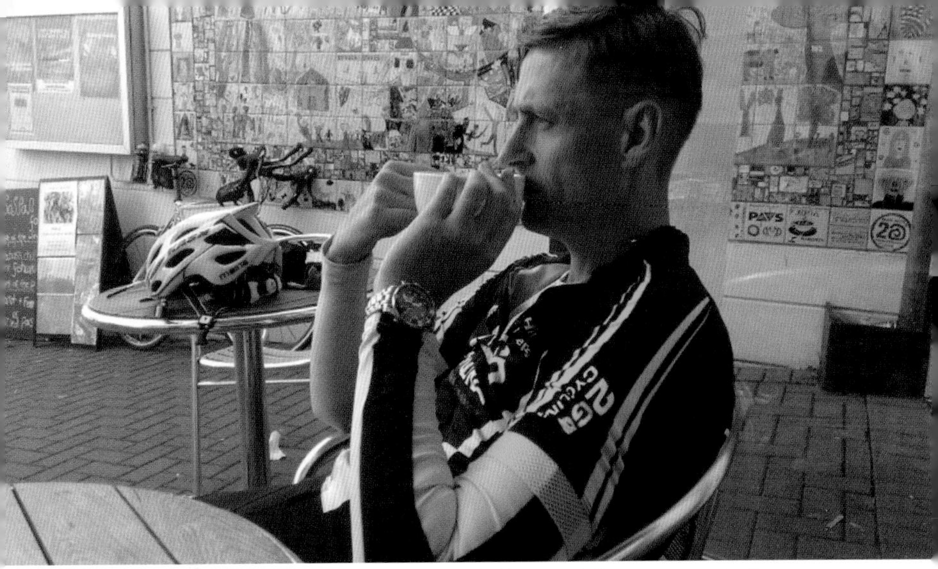

Contemplating failure after completing the 'hilly bit' of the Ironman Wales cycle course

Not contemplating failure as I cross the line at the Ocean Lava Wales Triathlon

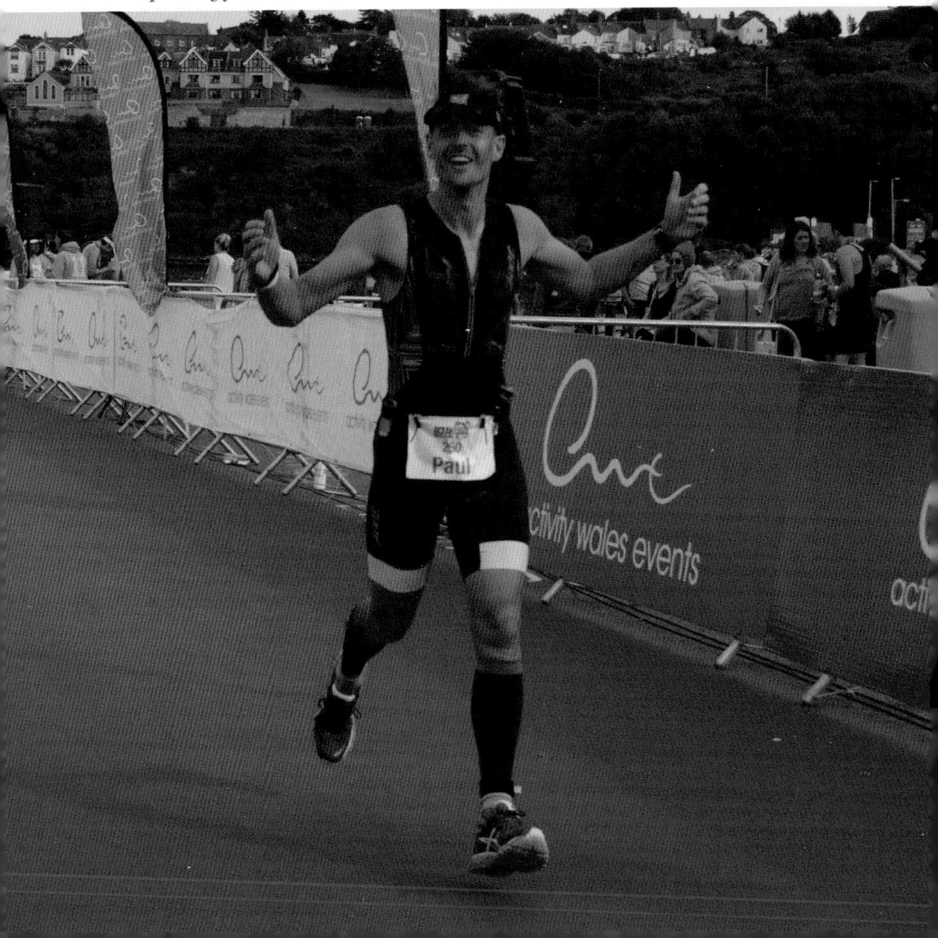

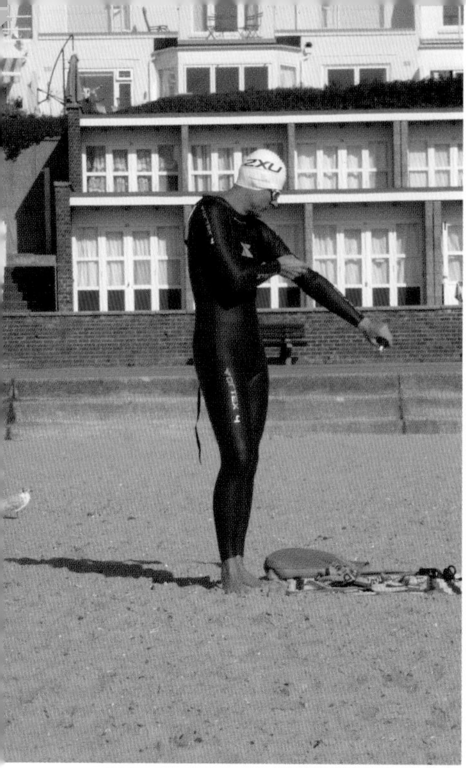

Preparing for a sea swim at a sunny Sandbanks, Bournemouth

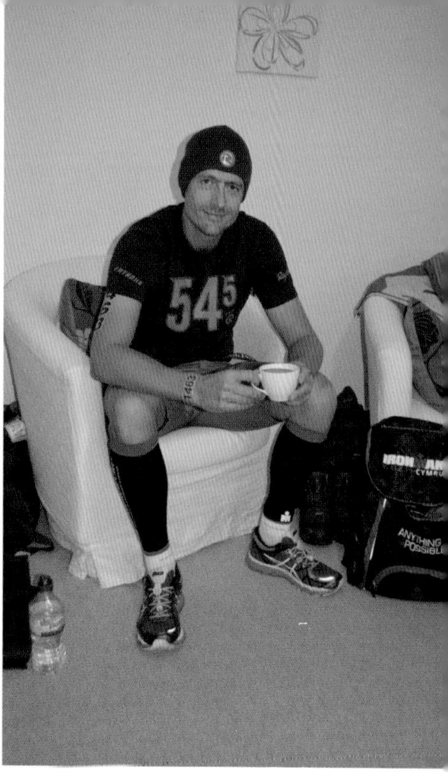

Relaxed and ready to go on race morning

Going to have to start swimming soon, entering the water at Ironman Wales

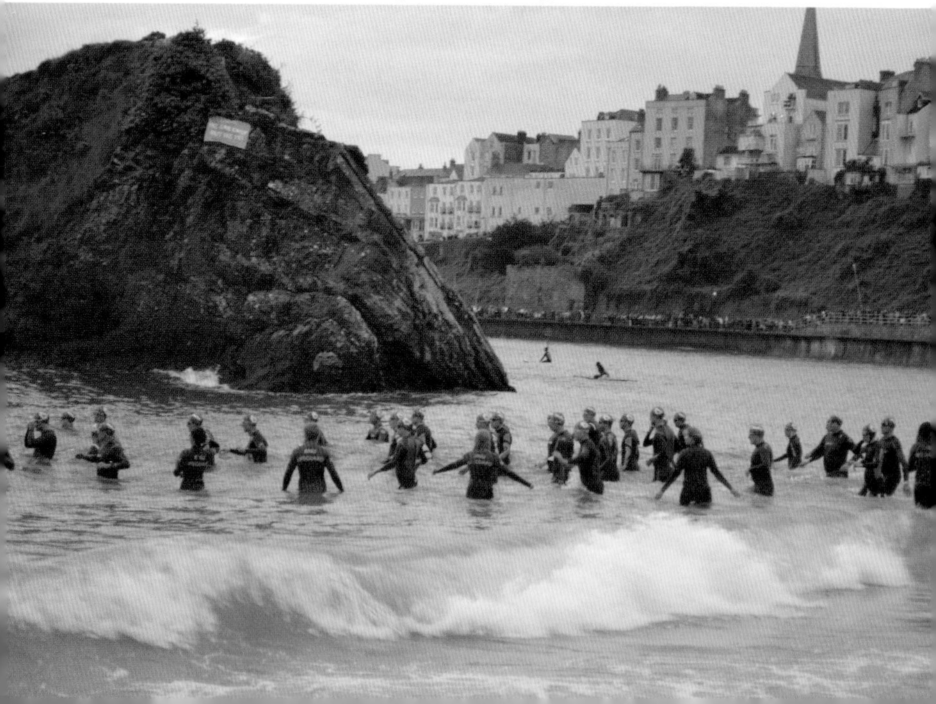

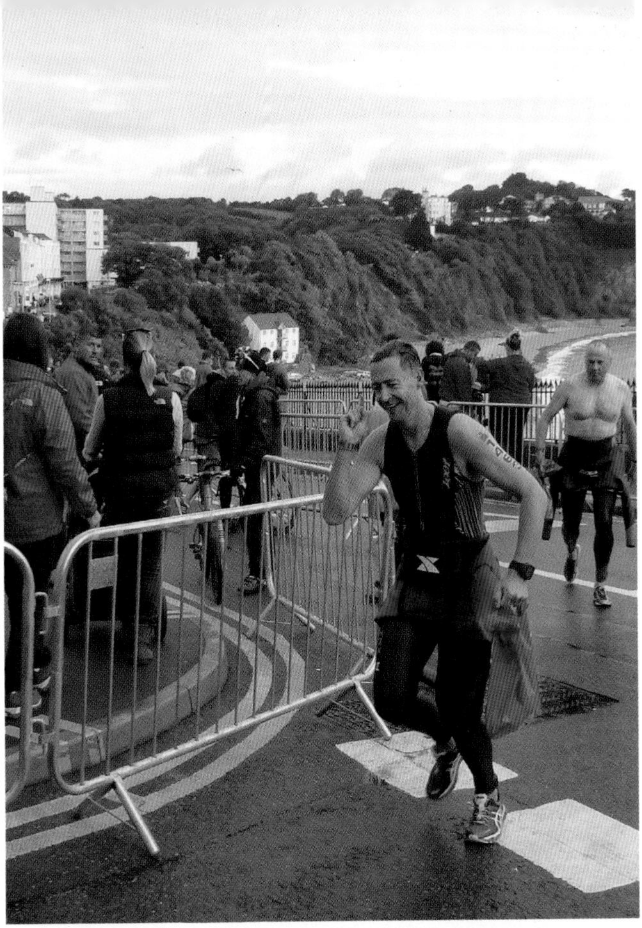

Swim to bike transition, very relieved to get that swim out of the way

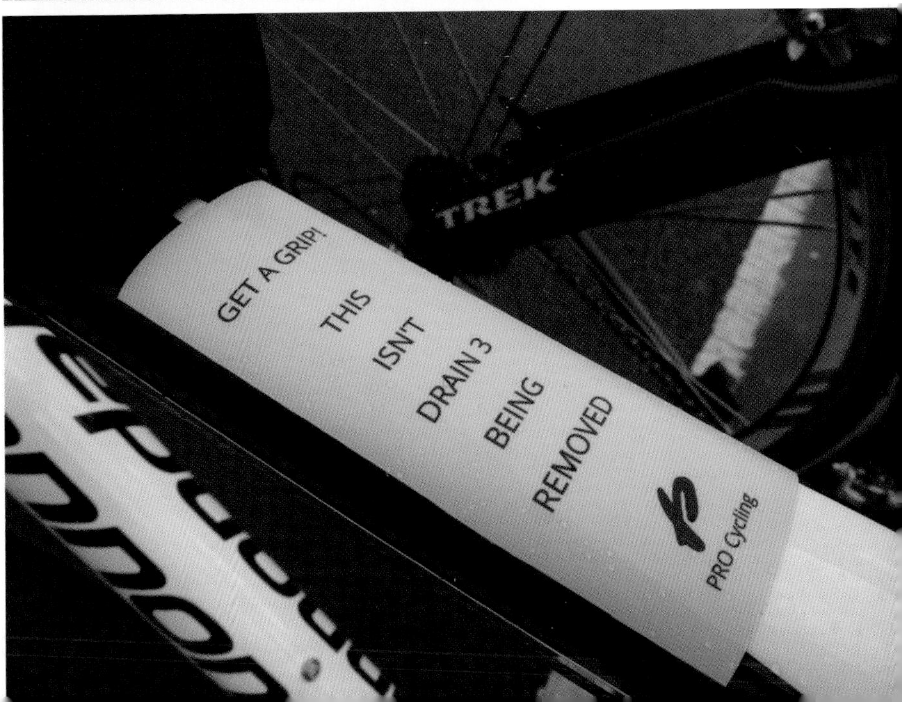

A bit of race motivation. It turned out to be the truth, just

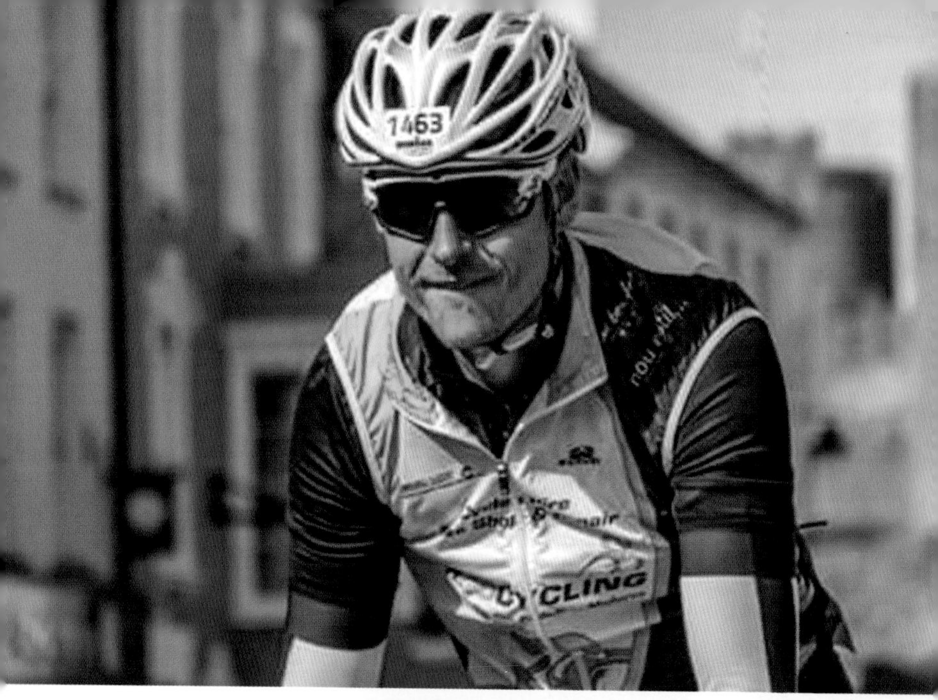

Still feeling fresh and powering down Pembroke High Street

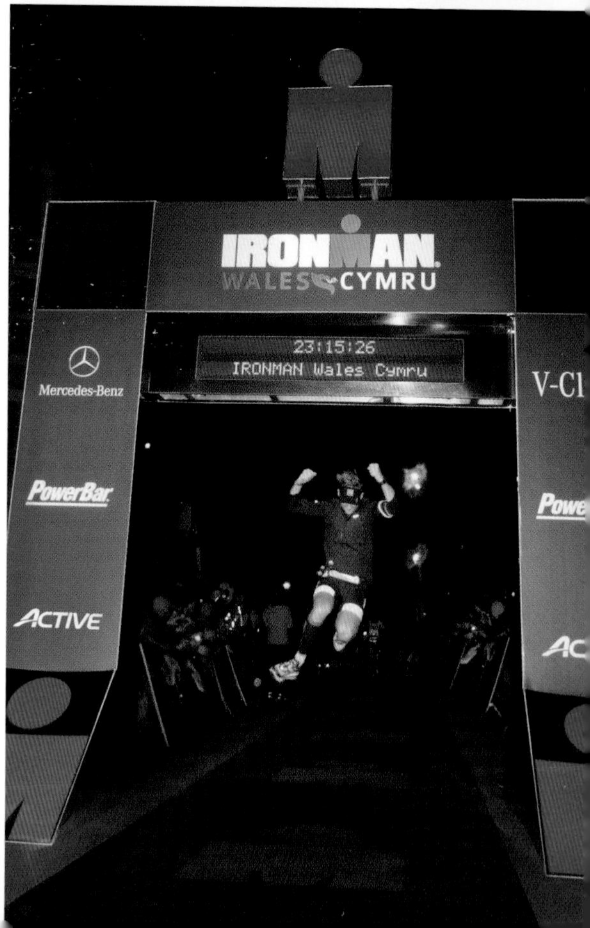

Paul, you are an Ironman!

was visibly thinner and, rooting around in my wardrobe for something to wear, I found that literally none of my clothes fitted me anymore. I had gone from a size large to a very loose medium. The weight off my chest and back was the most noticeable – I looked like Chris Froome without the veiny legs.

Every cloud has a silver lining though, and I knew that carrying all that weight around the Ironman course would have been hard work. I couldn't imagine that I would have lost that much weight through exercise alone, so the skeleton that stared back at me from the mirror was the perfect frame on which to hang an endurance athlete's body, even if it was a bit crooked.

This athlete needed to start somewhere and it began with slow daily walks around the estate from the house. On my first outing I made it about 100 metres down the road before I felt so weak and sore that, after a couple of minutes clinging to a railing, I had to turn back through fear of coming up short and being found lying in a neighbour's garden when they got home from work. Back in the safety of the house, I collapsed on the sofa, exhausted.

I persevered with it, and over the next few days I progressed so quickly that by the end of that first week I was walking about three-quarters of a mile and doing a full circuit of the estate. It was hard going though, and I was getting back just as knackered as I was when I finished the Drogo Ten in November, so I didn't exactly feel great. The training programme I was hoping to follow called for exercise six days a week. It started with 15-minute bouts of running, cycling and swimming and built from there. I had the time to plan a training diary and my first full week's training was duly planned for the middle of January, giving me just five weeks to get myself into good enough shape to finish it.

Three weeks post-operation and my first real physical challenge manifested itself in the shape of some unexpected nerve awakenings. The worst of the pain from the operation had now subsided and I was just left numb from the ribs down to my hips, but in a matter of a few hours I went from a constant but manageable dull ache to feeling every little movement of my bowels and it felt like a ball of snakes spinning around inside me. These sensations were accompanied by painful contractions which would bend me double during the day and at night I would wake up in agony. I sat in bed clutching my knees to my chest and would rock gently for hours in the dark until it passed. Some days I would wonder if it would get any better at all and what life would be like if this was as good as it got. It was a horrible thought and a sobering one when you consider people who live with chronic pain in their lives. I was hoping for a pretty normal life when everything settled down, but this was torture, I was swallowing paracetamol like it was going out of fashion.

Christmas was spent at my sister's and was a very low-key affair for me, the highlight being my first full dinner at the Christmas lunch. I ate one roast potato, two Brussels sprouts and one slice of turkey with a thimble of gravy over the top. I followed it up with a wafer thin slice of Viennetta ice cream. How things had changed from the fine dining experiences I was having just two months before.

The very worst night I endured during my recovery was on New Year's Eve when we went over to a party at Luigi's house. It was the first time I'd had a drink since my operation and overdoing the buffet by two cocktail sausages, alongside the three bottles of Peroni I drank, did something terrible to my insides. I woke up in agony at about 3:00 in the morning with my bowels violently pulsing and waves of cramping washing across my abdomen. I was in so much pain that by four in the morning I was sitting sweating in the dark considering asking Maria to take me back to hospital. I sat tight and within the hour, much to my relief, the pain slowly began to subside and I eventually fell back to sleep.

The next day I decided to rein in my eating and drinking as I clearly wasn't ready for a return to anything like a normal diet. I was back at home but I couldn't kid myself that I was back to my old self, there was a lot of healing still to go.

We had a few days away for my birthday in Tenby and taking in the fresh air and the beaches definitely blew away the stuffy indoor cobwebs of the last few weeks and gave me another opportunity to recce some of the Ironman course, albeit from the inside of the car this time. I was still struggling with terrible cramping every time I ate, and after one pub lunch I was again left bent double clinging to an iron railing for dear life on my way back to the hotel. My recovery was going slower and was more painful than I had ever expected.

Getting back home and despite all my best intentions, I found myself nursing my first hangover of the year following a visit from my good friend Pete. I fully intended to restrain myself but two pints, a bottle of wine each and three large glasses of port meant that I wasn't going to avoid the inevitable. To understand the lack of control I exhibited, it's important to understand a bit about our relationship.

I met Pete years ago when we both worked together at the local water company. I was an area manager and Pete was on the new graduate intake. We only had a passing acquaintance in the first few months as we didn't work directly together, but a local beer festival was the catalyst which would cement our now long-standing boozy friendship. It transpired that we were the only two from work who fancied going so we took a day off and made it our mission to get there early and sample pretty much every barrel of ale and cider on offer.

Several blurry hours later we had somehow ended up taking ownership of a big shaggy dog attached to a length of string and a large bag of weed, and we had no idea what we were going to do with either. Fortunately we managed to negotiate a return of both by the end of the day but that crazy drunken afternoon started a lifelong friendship fuelled by ever increasing amounts of alcoholic excess. It went on like this for many years until, to the great relief of my liver, Pete moved abroad for work. We are still great mates and still enjoy a drink on the rare occasions we get a chance to meet up and that night was another of those rare occasions – I'd even go as far as to say that we took it easy.

Recovering from my hangover, it was time to think about how I was going to move on a stage from the bent-over geriatric I was currently impersonating to someone at least contemplating doing a structured fitness programme. I got my diary back out and started sketching out a plan for the next few weeks as that five-day exercise week was looming, so I needed to ratchet things up a notch.

Swimming felt like it was out for a few more weeks as the 12-inch scar on my abdomen was still very tight and I still couldn't really straighten up properly. This meant that I'd have to concentrate on my running and cycling, so I fixed my bike to the turbo trainer in the garage and did my first 20-minute spin. I took it easy and with every pedal stroke I could feel the tightness in my hips and back, but I was doing it and I didn't appear to be suffering too badly. In that 20 minutes I raised my heart rate for the first time and by the end of the session I could feel it thumping away in my chest and temples. As I climbed stiffly off the bike and wiped my sweaty brow, I felt good as this was the first time I had done some proper exercise since the operation, and it felt like real progress.

I followed this up with my first jog a few days later. It was a chilly day and I wrapped up well against the cold. The plan was to make it all the way around the estate so I went off gently but my legs started complaining straight from the moment I stepped out of the door. I felt incredibly weak but surprisingly I wasn't in any great pain which was a very good sign. My lungs were itching from the cold air as I sucked in big gulps trying to get some much-needed oxygen into my legs. I could feel my useless abs shaking with each stride but I got through it and had managed to jog for a very gentle mile. I considered going further but thought better of it and turned back for home – this was not the time to take chances. I had been told that there was a real risk of a hernia this soon after the operation, so if I didn't want another operation later in the year, I needed to look after myself.

That weekend Maria and I went out for our first proper bike ride. It was bitterly cold but dry and we managed an hour or so around the flat parts of town. The thing I noticed the most on that ride was how wobbly I had become on the bike. I had no core strength whatsoever and I found myself swaying and wobbling around as I pedalled. I had no chance of keeping up with Maria, so rolled it out and simply enjoyed the sensation of being out in the fresh air. I was glad to find I still had a love for the bike considering how much time I would need to be spending on it over the next few months.

I reached the end of that week still in one piece and was as ready as I'd ever be to start my first five-day exercise week, starting the following Monday. I was now also a pro at administering my blood-thinning injections and with the last couple of phials left rattling in the fridge, I would be pleased to see the back of that unpleasant daily ritual. My legs were covered in tiny bruises and lumps and bumps, but at least I knew that I'd be able to prepare myself for a career in professional cycling if I ever needed to.

Slow and Steady

IT WAS now mid-January. I was coming up to two months post-surgery and was about to embark on my first five-day training week. I was going to approach it steadily as I was still experiencing quite a lot of discomfort and physically I was still exhausted most of the time. The fear of a hernia was helping to hold me back from pushing on too quickly, but I was also aware that I only had eight months until the event so I couldn't sit back too much; training through some level of discomfort was unfortunately going to be the reality for me to reach the numbers I would need to complete the race within the time limits.

I was aware before the operation that I would have a long way to go from a very low starting point, but this knowledge was spurring me on to get better and I knew it would improve my overall health in the long run. My training plan needed some refining, so I set myself some milestones and began writing a training diary in which

I recorded everything from my workouts to my thoughts and moods. I've mentioned before that I love a good list and this was the perfect way to organise myself and see my goals laid out in front of me. The first thing I wrote in it, in big black letters, was the date of the Ironman – 13 September 2015.

I had never completed a triathlon before and I wanted to do at least one before the main event, so I started scouring the internet for triathlons in Wales to replicate the difficulty and conditions of the Ironman. Two stood out for me and were timed perfectly for my training.

Since the Ironman came to Tenby, lots of events have sprung up in Wales and many try to maximise the interest in them by aligning themselves with recommended training plans for the Ironman. The two I had chosen were the Ocean Lava Middle Distance Wales Triathlon in Fishguard and the Long Course Weekend in Tenby.

First up would be the Long Course Weekend. The event consists of the three separate triathlon disciplines over three days of a weekend in early July. The courses for the sea swim and the bike follow the Ironman route and the run, held on the Sunday, follows a different but equally challenging and hilly course. The main event is the full Long Course consisting of the full distance swim, bike and run with all the times added together for a finishing time under 17 hours. All the events have their individual cut-off times and you need to achieve all three to win the coveted Golden Long Course Medal.

In addition to the full event, you can complete a half-distance swim, one of two shorter bike rides and either a ten-kilometre or a half-marathon run. I booked the

1.2-mile sea swim for Maria and myself, and the 68-mile bike ride(a single full loop of the Ironman Wales course) and the half-marathon just for myself. Tom had confirmed he would do the same and I booked camping for all of us at a nearby site for the weekend. The first milestone had been laid down and now for the second.

The Ocean Lava Wales Triathlon in Fishguard was perfectly placed six weeks before Ironman Wales. It consisted of two events, both starting together from the quay in Fishguard harbour. A sprint distance consisting of a 750-metre sea swim, followed by a 13-mile bike leg and a three-mile run. The middle distance race was a 1.2-mile sea swim, a 56-mile bike ride and a half-marathon. The bike and run legs are hilly and nicely replicate the Ironman course. I booked the sprint for Maria and the middle distance for myself,. We also booked a week's holiday in Wales before the race to acclimatise and do some last-minute training.

My targets were set, so all I had to do now was improve in steady increments to hit them, no worries there then. What was worrying me though was the swim leg. I hadn't been back in the water since the operation and after making a decent attempt to cure my aquaphobia last year it had crept back with a vengeance. I wasn't physically ready for swimming but I could already feel myself putting it back and even avoiding thinking about it. This mental battle was definitely going to be my biggest – the cut-off time for both swims I had chosen was a worrying one hour. The Ironman swim has a cut-off of two hours 20 minutes so although both were half the distance, they were ten minutes shorter in the equivalent time limit. I would need to use the embarrassing thought of missing the cut to give me the necessary kick up the arse to get back in the water.

The following Monday it was time to put up, shut up and begin what would be the official start of my training year. If all went to plan I would be training six days a week from the start of my Iron fit programme, in just one month's time. So it was definitely time to get in the habit no matter how short the efforts were.

I started with a 20-minute spin on the turbo trainer and I felt good and not too sore. I was slowly starting to adapt, so Tuesday I went for a very gentle jog around the estate. Running was still difficult as the constant jiggling and jarring motion of it really pulled on my scar; I was slow and tentative but I got around. I felt tight afterwards, so thought it would be a good idea to do some core stretching and a ten-minute easy pilates routine I found on the internet.

The next morning I woke up regretting it badly; I'd clearly overdone it on the abs. I was pulled down tightly as I tried to get out of bed and it took ten minutes of gentle stretching and a warm shower to stand myself upright. I had planned my first swim that day but decided against it. I was disappointed as I knew I needed to get into that bloody pool, but somewhere deep down I was still secretly relieved that I could avoid it for another day. This conflict of interests was troubling and I couldn't make those excuses for much longer or I would start to damage my chances. I couldn't understand why it was so hard to motivate myself when I knew what was at stake. Thursday was better but I still felt sore, so it was another day of enforced rest. I therefore had two more sessions to do over the weekend to hit that five-day target.

Saturday I went for another gentle jog and managed one and a half miles. I got back feeling fine so the two days' rest had obviously done me some good. On the Sunday we dressed up against the cold and went out on the bikes for a one-hour, 12-mile spin around the local villages. I got back and congratulated myself for achieving the five-day goal even though it looked a little different to what I'd initially envisaged.

I vowed to go to the pool the next day and packed my bag in readiness. There were to be no excuses this time. I didn't need to rush as I could go to my usual 20m pool attached to a local school and join the pensioners in their mid-morning open swim session. As I walked through the doors that familiar warmth and the waft of chlorine enveloped me and I felt a bit sick. Why was I so nervous? I just couldn't understand it. I changed quickly and rinsed off under the poolside shower. As I showered I noticed an old lady bobbing in the pool who was peeping at me over the side through her tinted goggles. Who could blame her, I thought to myself, but then I realised as I followed her eyes that she was looking at my scar. Dressed in my trunks, it was an impressive sight. A long crooked purple rope diving down from my ribcage into my low-cut swimming jammers with neat rows of staple marks on either side. It was flanked by some equally impressive angry-looking puncture wounds. It looked all the stranger for the fact that I no longer had a belly button and had clearly been sewn up a bit lopsided. My hand instinctively went to cover it but I stopped myself. That scar was a reminder to me of what I had been through and I definitely had nothing to hide or be ashamed of, so I wore it with pride from that day on. It also served a very useful purpose as a nice little silent excuse for onlookers to explain why I was so shit at swimming, just coming back from surgery and all that.

I sat on the edge of the pool, took a deep breath and lowered myself in. It was chilly and goose pimples erupted over me.

I left my pull buoy on the side, put on my goggles and nose plug, and dived straight down into the water. I swam a few metres under the water which felt surprisingly good, then came up and started to swim a few gentle lengths of breaststroke. I could feel my abs tightly pulling as I reached forwards with my stroke, but with each stroke the discomfort became less and less, and was nothing at this stage of my recovery that I couldn't handle. I swam for 30 minutes, half breaststroke and half front crawl, and even swam four lengths of crawl without the pull buoy between my legs. As I walked back out of the doors 45 minutes later, I was chuffed to pieces that I had broken the back of it – it could only be up from here because that was a poor swim to be honest. I promised myself a swim at least once a week until the programme started proper.

If anything was going to derail my Ironman dream it would likely be one of the two long-standing injuries I had been contending with since my mid-20s. The first and possibly more serious was the problem I had with my right shoulder. Since my days of goalkeeping for my local Sunday league football team I had suffered with bouts of rotator cuff pain. The rotator cuff is the joint at the top of your shoulder coming from the collar bone. Our team were so bad that it must have been an overuse injury from all the diving around I had to do. I only had to sleep heavily on it for it to become painful and sometimes I couldn't even raise my arm above my head to wash my hair. I hadn't thrown a ball overarm for near-on 20 years, as this would always strain the joint and put me out of action for weeks at a time. On occasion it would become so painful that the muscles would bind up and I would need to see a chiropractor; one time I even resorted to acupuncture to loosen it up. It would flare up at least once a year, and if it came on a week before the Ironman it would be an absolute showstopper. The concern was how it would fare with all the swimming I was going to be doing in the run-up – it was only ever going to go one of two ways and one of them didn't bear thinking about.

The second injury was my true Achilles heel, both in fact. Any form of exercise made them ache. I'd had physiotherapy twice before to relieve the symptoms but they were knotted, scarred and prone to bouts of chronic pain. This injury came about in my early 30s when I played a lot of five-a-side football with my work team. I'd wake up in the mornings after a match and dance about on tiptoes like a ballerina until they had warmed up sufficiently to allow me to get on with my day, and by the end of the week they just about loosened up enough to allow me to rush out and play another football match. I researched the symptoms on the internet and read 'these injuries are suffered mostly by males in their late 20s or early 30s who think they can play sport at the same intensity as when they were in their early 20s without warming up.' Well that was definitely me then and I was still paying for it all these years later.

Over the next few weeks I slowly upped my exercise times and intensities. I was now eating more and my bowel movements were improving all the time. It's amazing what a nice firm poo can do for your well-being when you wondered, at one point, whether you would be able to venture more than five minutes away from a toilet in your life again. This was a real plus for someone daft enough to be thinking about completing a 17-hour endurance event.

I plunged straight into the ten-week build phase with a swim, a solid 30 minutes of sustained front crawl with the comfort blanket of my pull buoy tucked firmly between my legs. I knew that I was overusing it but figured that it replicated the buoyancy I got from wearing a wetsuit, so that wasn't going to be a big problem. The work I had put in meant I had been exceeding the starting points for each discipline in the initial programme, but the big difference was that I was now exercising six times a week and sometimes twice a day. This upping of the intensity was a big difference but the results started to show quickly. I was stronger and more controlled in all the disciplines and thankfully still remained injury free.

It was now March and I was already considering going back to work; the police are a fantastic employer when it comes to looking after their staff and I was looked after excellently. There was no expectation of me returning so soon, but I was told to take three months off while I was at the hospital and they were right. After three months the tiredness had passed, and although I wasn't 100 per cent I was a lot stronger and quite capable of doing a day's work. A backroom position had come up and I had been offered it. It was a good fit for me as I was in no position to be wrestling villains just yet, but I was very happy to be back doing my bit and driving a desk. They wanted me to go back part-time initially but I was happy to jump straight back in full-time. I was getting bored at home and was looking forward to having some company around me during the day again.

I started back with a two-week residential training course in Portishead near Bristol, which was essential for my new role. I figured that I could take my running gear and get in some evening jogs along the coastline. The downside was that the course started with a day-long exam and practical assessment which was a pass or fail for progression to the full course the following week. Even though my body had been getting plenty of exercise, I couldn't say the same for my brain which really struggled to get the synapses firing. It was an exhausting rude awakening but I got through it with a pass and into the second week. The only real downside of being back at work was that my swims would now have to be at six in the morning when I had to share the pool with elite swimmers and the assorted Ironmen who always stalked the leisure centre that early in the day. There is nothing like a ridiculously early start and being forced to the side of the pool because you dare not even look in the lanes, let alone attempt to swim in them. I hope at least some of them noticed the scar and took a bit of pity on me.

I fitted some aero bars on to my bike at the beginning of the year and had now just begun to experiment with them – aero bars are those things that you can fix to the handlebars of your bicycle with elbow cups and long bars for gripping which hold you into a tucked-in and aerodynamic position on the bike. I had started to use them for short periods on the turbo trainer to get used to the more forward and lower position they force you into. They really hurt my abs and back at first and I wasn't yet convinced about the advantages for me.

One thing I was convinced about though was the benefit of having a proper bike fit where a professionally trained fitter adjusts your bike to the optimal position for your riding and body shape. The benefits are more comfort, better power delivery and a reduced risk of injury. The year before when I got my first road bike, I went rushing off for my first long ride and had my saddle positioned way too high. I ruined both my Achilles tendons for weeks after that, so I knew it wasn't a gimmick.

I opted for a fully scientific fitting with computer measurements and sensors positioned on all my joints to track the angles. It wasn't cheap but I figured if I was going to be spending ten to 12 hours on my bike every week then it would be worth it. Two hours and £100 later I walked out with my saddle raised by all of about one centimetre. Oh well, at least I now had all the measurements if I ever needed a new bike.

One thing I had been toying with was whether to shave my legs or not. Because of all the exercise, I was now spending a lot of time in very tight-fitting Lycra and the Wookie-like legs that were sprouting out from under the shorts weren't very flattering. I knew I'd be ridiculed for it at work but it's what the pros did, so what the hell. One evening as I was about to jump into the shower I nabbed Maria's razor and without telling her I got to work. It took ages to hack back the bushes and I was a prune by the time I got out, but after applying some moisturiser I stood in front of the mirror and admired my silky smooth pins. It's surprising what a de-fuzz can do for muscle definition, and with arms like pipe cleaners at least I could now show off the guns I was starting to develop.

If you look a pro you feel pro and that's a real confidence boost and another small step towards making an Ironman out of me, although afterwards I did need to become familiar with the art of exfoliating following a nasty bout of ingrown hairs – who knew the problems that women have to put up with?

It was an exciting week because my new mountain bike was also being delivered. This was the most expensive bicycle I'd ever owned and was a real beast. Long-travel suspension and big fat tyres on oversized wheels made it a real go-anywhere machine. I had wanted a new one since the suspension had bottomed out badly on my old bike on that lad's weekend in Wales, nearly throwing me off into the trees as a consequence. The cancer sympathy ticket was still valid, so another treat was definitely in order and I cashed it in.

That weekend I met Luigi at the Bracknell Forest trail centre to give it its maiden ride out. We stuck to the easier blue trail which was a rolling single-track path through the forest with some climbing as well as some nice sweeping descents. My fitness from the near-daily sessions was starting to show and I was pleased to see that I was faring better than my friend as we wound our way around the course. Training on my own meant I had very little to gauge my improving fitness against, so any sessions with friends really showed me where I was in terms of progress. A few years before he would have been kicking my arse, I had no doubt about that.

As my long runs approached the ten-kilometre mark, I was having to start thinking about nutrition. I had read of the importance of fuelling during an Ironman due to the long nature and high-calorie burn of the event. If you got your fuelling wrong you would fail without question, no matter how fit you were. I read that it was often referred to as an eating race as much as anything else.

It was also important to start to train the body to absorb nutrition while you exercised. This wasn't a given and you had to build it up over a long time, alongside your physical training, so I brought mountains of energy bars and energy gels in different flavours and began to experiment. A hundred calories every 20 minutes is a good guide as the body can only absorb around 300 calories an hour anyway, which equated to a single sachet of gel or half a Snickers bar or something similar. Energy drinks can also provide the calories needed alongside the required hydration, and some people will do a whole race on fluids alone.

Another significant milestone was achieved when I ran my first ten kilometres in under one hour. I was training within heart rate zones, so I was impressed that I achieved it without my heart rate going through the roof. There was still a long way to go but what I was doing appeared to be working. I still had to manage my pain with a lot of paracetamol and I got very sore if I overdid things, but it was a good indicator for me to stick to the plan and take things nice and steadily.

I got to May and as the weather was warming up it was time to literally dive in and get to grips with some open-water swimming. It was without a doubt still my weakest discipline and the one I feared the most. The training plan called for very prescribed sessions of swimming involving different drills like swimming with legs only using swim fins to develop strength, but when I tried it I just got a cramp in my hamstrings and barely made it to the side of the pool without being hooked out by the lifeguard. After much deliberation I decided that I would just swim for as far and long as I could each session in front crawl and, by a process of sheer attrition, I would build enough strength and technique to get me through the 2.4-mile swim. That number was still frightening me but only by doing it would that fear go away. So on the opening day I took myself back down to the lake.

The cold murky waters got me after only a few hundred metres and I was already gasping for breath between strokes. I could feel that old panic slowly rising inside me, so I stopped and rolled on to my back. I had an asthma inhaler up my wetsuit sleeve, so I took a couple of deep puffs and looked around. The water was cold but the sky was blue and the evening sun sparkled across it, and it struck me that there were far worse places to be on a Tuesday evening. I took a moment to relax then rolled over to put my head under the water and let the buoyancy of my wetsuit float my legs up behind me. I stared down into the weeds as I blew out my breath in a gentle stream of bubbles. I watched the fish swimming effortlessly below me for a few seconds before slowly starting to rotate my arms. I felt the catch of the water as my strokes began to propel me forward and used my legs sparingly, allowing them to float behind me as I went on to swim two full laps of the lake, which was around 1,500m. I went on to do at least two lake sessions each week from then on right up until the Ironman. It was a big relief to be out of the pool and I felt I could do my own thing in the lake away from the prying eyes of the lifeguards and expert swimmers who I always seemed to be getting in the way of.

With all my signed-up events including a sea swim, this was another element I needed to practise. My first sea swim came one sunny day at Sandbanks in Bournemouth. Maria sunbathed as I suited up and went in for a planned one-kilometre swim down the beach and back. The buoyancy of the salt water was unreal and I felt like I was flying as I set off down the beach 20 metres out into a calm but gently bobbing sea. As I reached about 400 metres I realised I was starting to feel quite unwell. I think I had swallowed a lot of seawater as I breathed and I started burping loudly and retching under the water. I thought I was going to be sick so I swam to the shore so I could stand up. As my feet hit the sand and I stood up I wobbled giddily around as I retched up a mouthful of my breakfast. I was completely seasick from a combination of the bobbing sea, the salty water and the buoyancy of my swimming wetsuit.

I got myself together, wiped the tears out from the inside of my goggles and turned back towards where I could see Maria lying on the beach in the distance, and began swimming again. I felt weak and sick and each time I lifted my head to sight the tiny speck that was Maria in the distance, she didn't seem to be getting any bigger no matter how hard I swam. I realised that I was now swimming against the tide which must have carried me away on the way out – no wonder I was swimming like a champ. I eventually got back to her exhausted, pale and sickly. I was shocked how long it had taken me to swim just 800 metres – at that pace I would have been struggling to make the swim time limits for my events. This was something I was determined to be well inside of and I didn't need the extra stress of missing the cut on top of everything else I had to contend with. My pool and lake swimming times were pretty consistent and would have me finishing the full distance in around one hour 45 to one hour 50. I was slow but I was happy that I would have at least 30 minutes to spare, but that day I would have been lucky to finish at all.

I would need to dig a little bit deeper to get the swimming done and needed to plan in a lot more sea swimming to get used to the different conditions. I hadn't yet had to contend with any waves or swell and the Ironman Wales had some truly horrendous swimming conditions over the years. It wouldn't be good enough to just hope for a calm day.

As the weeks went by my body was holding up and the six days a week were starting to work their magic. During June I was up to three laps of the lake and swimming 2,500 metres at least once a week. My long rides were touching 60 miles and my weekly long runs were now up to two hours and ten miles in length. I was also smashing my ten-kilometre personal best every week on my speed runs. I was still constantly sore and the night-time cramps were stubbornly not easing, but I was getting confident that I could make the grade for my first triathlon challenge at the Long Course Weekend in Tenby.

Looking back, I couldn't believe how far I had come in the six months since my first painful steps out of our front door on those cold January mornings. Any sensible person would probably have given themselves a pat on the back at that point and taken the plaudits before getting on with their life. I, on the other hand, was the fool who wasn't even halfway into my journey yet, so it was a bloody good job I was still smiling even if occasionally it was through gritted teeth.

The Long Course Weekend – Part 1

I'D KEPT myself motivated as the training ramped up but I think there may have been a bit of fear in the mix as I really needed a good performance at the Long Course Weekend to give me some confidence. I had plugged away through the pain and some truly miserable winter weather and I was now desperate for a sporting achievement to show for it.

When you are doing the exact same training programme as a friend it's very difficult not to get competitive with each other. Tom and I had been dissecting every step of every session and the levels of banter were spiralling ever higher as the event got closer. We had been out together on a couple of long bike rides during the previous few weeks, and although I had the makings of him on the first ride by stretching him out on the hills the second time around was a much tighter affair as he was pushing the pace on right from the start. I had to maintain a full-on poker face and by the end I was barely hanging on to his wheel when we got back to his house for a celebratory fried breakfast.

The swim was no contest; Tom was a good swimmer and I was not. He was doing the full 2.4-mile swim at the Long Course Weekend and I was still fretting about making the cut-off on the half distance. It didn't help matters when he would come into work and tell me he had been swimming like a Viking during his morning pool session. Who knew what that even meant, but the thought of sharing a lane with him in his tight trunks while he was going full Viking was quite terrifying.

The bike leg would be a lot more even. We would be riding together in a group of three, the third member being another mate of mine who was joining us for the 68-mile Wales Sportive. We planned to do the circuit in under five hours, which would be around the pace required for the Ironman. As it was a sportive, we had the advantage of being able to slipstream behind each other to share the effort. This was a luxury banned in Ironman events which are in effect solo time trials. I had been training quite hard on the bike and had even included some epic cycles to work. I would leave the house at six in the morning and cycle the 23 very hilly country miles to the office and then cycle the same hilly route back home. I was confident I could cover the distance and had a fuelling plan sorted, so I envisaged no real problems.

The half-marathon was going to be a tough one to call, as Tom had been playing his running down in the weeks leading up to the event. He'd been droning on about a sore knee and there was also something wrong with his arse, meaning that he had apparently missed some sessions, but I wasn't convinced that he wasn't just keeping his powder dry and was secretly planning on running me into the ground. I had trained well and with my long runs now up to ten miles I could sustain a pace to finish in around two hours ten on the flat, but this course was very hilly and would probably involve some speed walking up the steepest hills. My previous best for a half-marathon was two hours 19 minutes, some three years previously. Tom's personal best was two hours six, so this was going to be the time to beat.

We were staying at a large campsite near to Tenby and travelled down late on the Thursday evening after work. Tom and his family, with their newborn baby, were travelling down at the same time and were slightly ahead of us. As we crossed into Pembrokeshire around eleven in the evening, I got a call saying that they had arrived but the security wouldn't let him in as we didn't have a reservation. My heart sank. Bloody hell, I was sure I booked it months ago. Maria was trying to look through old emails on my phone to find the reservation as we drove. In the meantime they had been left at the gate with a newborn baby and another over-tired child whilst the security guard went off to the office to double check the paperwork. They were fully booked and it wasn't looking promising. After much discussion on the phone and a lot of swearing by me, it transpired that I had booked the correct dates but when I phoned up to add an extra night to the booking the agent had changed the whole booking to the month before in error. Eventually the over-cautious security guard showed them some pity and lifted the gate so that they could be shown to a double pitch where we could set up camp.

The next morning the sun was shining and Tom and I were sent packing off to the reception to complain. We were very British about it all, accepting the duty manager's apology and coming away with nothing other than the 'luxury' pitch we had been dumped on the night before, despite Maria insisting that we should have asked for a free holiday or our money back. She wasn't happy.

The Long Course Weekend is a big event for the town and it attracts thousands of competitors to all three of the events and the full Long Course itself. The bunting is hung out across the town and large crowds of spectators come out to support the athletes. We walked into town and weaved our way through the crowded streets to the signing-in area to collect our timing chips and race numbers. When you get your hands on these things it all starts to feel a bit real and the pre-race nerves start to jangle. The swim was that evening from the North Beach, so we had some time to walk down to the harbour and view the course.

From an elevated position on the clifftop you can see the whole swim course laid out in front of you. The start line was being set up and the two large buoys that mark the corners of the triangular swim circuit were bobbing gently in a calm and shimmering sea. We hoped that the conditions would stay that way for the event in a few hours' time. The most unnerving thing about the scene was the huge barrel jellyfish washed up along the shoreline – these have been a feature of the Welsh coastline for a few years now and are quite a sight to see. I wasn't looking forward to bumping into one of those half a mile out in the bay. Tom reckoned any he encountered on the way around he would eat for energy.

I'd managed to swim a mile in the sea before the event but had found it very difficult – seasickness seemed to be my biggest issue when I spent a long time bobbing in the ocean. I was convinced in my mind that I could make the one hour cut-off, but it wasn't a given if there was a strong tide to swim against and I'd also not swam in such close proximity to so many others during a mass start either. There would be about 1,500 swimmers taking to the water all at the same time and the thrashing and kicking would be a problem unless I hung back, but by doing that I would burn more precious minutes which I couldn't afford to waste, so my tactics would need to be spot on when that gun went off.

I knew the event was well supported but I was surprised as we walked around the corner and were confronted with a huge crowd of competitors and spectators. The clifftops make a perfect amphitheatre for a large crowd to watch the event from and it was packed. We had to shuffle our way through the crowds to make our way down the steep steps and on to the beach. Just as we'd hoped, the sea was still calm and the sun was shining. It looked like perfect conditions to me.

There was a real buzz about the place and you could feel the anticipation in the air. At the water's edge we pulled on our wetsuits and had time for a quick dip in the sea to adjust to the temperature. The water felt cold and I took a couple of extra puffs on my inhaler as I felt my chest tighten when the coldness washed into my wetsuit.

I hid my inhaler by the foot of a crowd control barrier on the beach and took my place on the start line. Tom had pushed further towards the front to get a good start and Maria and I hung back towards the rear of the pack to avoid the worst of the pushing and kicking in the mass start. There was a sea of white swim caps in front of us as the countdown began for the start.

As the gun went off with a bang and fireworks were launched across the bay, my mouth went dry and my heart started to pound. This was really it, this was the first time in my life that my swimming was going to be tested and with the Ironman at stake I couldn't afford to fail. I gave Maria a quick hug and a smile and we started to shuffle forwards as the crowd of swimmers moved towards the water. I pulled my goggles down and adjusted them – the last thing I needed was an eyeful of salty water right at the start. The crowd in front began picking up pace as people started to enter the water and we found ourselves jogging as our feet hit the cold sea lapping at the sand.

I looked ahead to the first buoy floating in the distance and it looked a very long way away. I could see some of the elite swimmers were already halfway towards it and were swimming at an incredible pace. I knew that many of them would be lapping me about halfway around as they would be crossing the finish line at a similar time to me having swum twice as far.

I started to wade into the water and lost sight of Maria. I was on my own now, there were no hiding places here and it was time to get it done. I strode out to my waist and then my chest and had to tell myself to dive in and start swimming. I could feel my body resisting it, but there was no way I could walk all the way around. It was the nerves talking. I looked around me and saw that I was surrounded by some equally anxious people. It gave me some confidence that I wasn't alone out there and I went for it, the cold water hitting my face as I slid forwards into and under the water. The sea was murky from all the kicked-up sand and I lifted my head to sight the buoy before relaxing into my stroke. Within ten metres someone had drifted in front of me and kicked me full in the face. I swallowed a huge mouthful of salty water and started gagging and choking. In a moment of panic I tried to stand up but found I was already out of my depth and instantly sank under the water, swallowing another huge gulp of water. I doggy paddled to the surface and coughed hard to get my breath back, water splashing all around me as swimmers tried to get past.

I took a moment to compose myself but was feeling the urgency now. I didn't have time to mess about, I needed to get swimming. I lifted my legs behind me and felt the weight of somebody swimming over the back of them. My head went under again but this time I managed to gulp in a breath. I was starting to get annoyed now, there was plenty of room around us for people to pay a bit of attention and avoid these contacts. I kicked out with my feet and propelled myself forward. I felt contact with the swimmer that was trying to drown me and heard some swearing as he started to flounder in the water behind me. Sorry mate, it's every man for himself out here.

It felt good to be holding my own in the water and it gave me the confidence to hit my stroke and begin swimming at last. Swimming for me was a very mechanical and monotonous process and I needed to get into a rhythm to get my breathing right, and with that my pace would settle. I was starting to feel the water a bit more as the crowds thinned and I made my way out into the deeper water of the bay.

I constantly looked up to sight the first buoy as I didn't want to weave around and swim any further than I had to; I could see others to my left who seemed a long way off course already. As I approached the buoy I was struck by how big it was – it loomed over us and was quite intimidating in its size. The water was choppier here and there seemed to be some congestion as a group of swimmers all looked to cut the corner as tightly as they could.

I was soon up against the back of a crowd of around 20 bobbing white swim caps who had completely stopped swimming and were treading water and doggy paddling slowly around the buoy, and the pushing and dunking started again. I was pushed forcefully under the water as someone clattered into the back of me, but I had time to take a breath so there was no panic this time. I spotted a gap in the sea of heads and went for it. I couldn't get my legs up behind me to swim because of the crowd pressing down behind me but I made the gap, kicked my legs and swam away from the crowd. It felt like I'd overtaken a few people as I went away and that felt good.

I swam into clear water and found myself swimming on my own at last. There were lifeguards on paddle boards all over the course, so although this was the first time I had truly swam out of my depth in deep open water, I felt surprisingly calm and could relax and concentrate on getting it done. The second buoy, which was right up against the harbour wall, came quickly and I swam tightly around it unopposed as the congestion had now dispersed across the whole circuit. I was tiring a little but was still holding my form and as I lifted my head I could see the shore and the big inflatable finish line in the distance.

The last couple of hundred metres seemed to take an age to finish, and every time I lifted my head the beach just didn't seem to be getting any nearer. I had no idea of the time and was starting to worry that I may not make the one-hour cut-off; it was feeling like a very long time but I dared not break my stroke to look at my watch. I tried to up my pace but swallowed some more water as I started thrashing – the extra effort I was putting in was definitely not making me go any faster. I told myself to relax, keep to my own rhythm and just swim steadily for the beach.

As I neared the shore I thought I was close enough to touch the sand and stand up but as I went to stand I sank under the water, inhaling another huge mouthful of seawater. I was still well out of my depth and as I spluttered my way back to the surface I wasted another few precious seconds getting going again. I didn't learn from it as I tried to stand up again only a few metres later and once more I was splashing around trying to keep my head above the surface. It was a valuable lesson learnt to make sure I swam right until my hand touched the sand, one that I vowed to remember come Ironman race day.

I eventually managed to touch the bottom and rose with a wobble out of the water. I waded forwards and stumbled dizzily to my knees in the shallows and let out a huge burp from all the seawater I'd swallowed. I got back to my feet, took a deep breath and jogged up the beach towards the finish line. It was a great feeling to run through the cheering crowds and cross the line. I looked up and saw that the time was 50 minutes and 23 seconds – I couldn't believe it. That would see me a full 30 minutes ahead of the pace come the Ironman swim cut-off. I was chuffed to pieces and as a finishers' medal was hung around my neck I felt like I'd really achieved something significant. I'd battled and held my own in a mass start and I'd managed to compete in a swimming event for the first time in my life. I even managed to come in 127th out of 189 swimmers. I could barely believe that there were 62 worse swimmers than me in the entire world, let alone in Tenby that evening.

Maria had come in about four minutes before me and Tom smashed out the full swim in one hour and 22 minutes, an excellent time. Challenge number one was over and we were all feeling very happy if a little seasick. I was also feeling secretly relieved. I was at last able to banish some of those swimming demons that had been plaguing me and it felt good. It may have only been halfway but it was exactly where I needed to be. To cap it all off I didn't see a single jellyfish the whole way around.

The Long Course Weekend – Part 2

SAT HAVING breakfast in the sun, I was in a confident mood after the success of my swim, and although I knew the ride was going to be a tough one I was looking forward to it. The start was from a car park only about 500 metres from the campsite, so there was no stress about making our allotted start time of 9:30am.

Everything I had done in training and all the effort I had made was now starting to pay off. The cancer was pushed way into the back of my mind and I felt good, I was alive and literally kicking. In the middle of this weekend of sport I don't think I had ever felt such a sense of investment in something in my whole life. The lingering pain I felt from the operation was nothing in comparison to the achievement I was starting to feel regarding my fitness and my general health. Today I was going to take an equal share of the effort with two of my best friends, only eight months after my operation, and I was proud of that fact. It was also exciting, if a little frightening, knowing that I wasn't even halfway towards what I needed to achieve to become that Ironman. I was now well aware of the awesome difficulty of that challenge and it was that which was driving me on, giving me real purpose in my life and improving my recovery even further.

At the start line Tom and I sat on our crossbars soaking up some of the early morning sun as we watched the waves of starters roll off out of the car park and down the road. We were waiting for my good friend Muzz, the third member of our little team, to turn up so we could get the show on the road.

I have known Muzz since our first days in the police together, over 11 years at the time, and we are still good friends now; in fact, I have known him a little longer than that.

During the early stages of the recruitment process, way back in 2002, I was attending my medical examination and was shown into a typical white-walled waiting room with faded posters warning of the dangers of sexually-transmitted diseases sellotaped to the walls, a waft of disinfectant in the air and hard plastic chairs to sit on. As I looked around the room to get my bearings, I saw that there were only two chairs and one of them was taken by a short, stocky bloke with tightly cropped dark hair. He looked up, smiled and asked me how I was doing in a broad Geordie accent, and from that day forward we did every single stage of our recruitment and police training together and became very good friends as a result. He will probably kill me for calling him a Geordie and I will apologise to him for my lack of geographical knowledge of the north-east of England.

We already shared a taste for heavy metal and motorcycles and over the last few years had developed one for cycling long distances on uncomfortable bicycles. Muzz is ex-army and it often shows through in his character – he is a very straightforward bloke who doesn't overthink a challenge. If you pointed up a hill he would run up it and if you threw a ball he would fetch it with the enthusiasm of a Jack Russell. Head down and with the constitution of an ox, he will plough through any job until it's done, no fuss made and already moving on to the next, pretty much the complete opposite of me in fact. I would probably still be looking up the hill and asking why I needed to go up there and then looking at the ball and shaking my head, then would ask why you threw it away in the first place. He was just the man we needed to drag our sorry complaining arses around a hilly 70-miler when the going got tough.

'There he is.' Tom and Muzz had never met, so I pointed out his grinning face as it came weaving through the crowd towards us. I introduced them and we made our way straight to the start line and entered a penned-off area with about 30 other cyclists in the next wave of starters. There was a quick race briefing which basically reminded us all to stay on our side of the road and not to ride like an idiot, as it was an open-road course, and then we were off.

We pedalled away and let the crowd naturally thin out around us. Straight from the car park you hit a little hill as you turn left and then it's a glide away from the town until the first proper hill, only about half a mile further on from there.

It's very easy at the start of any event to get carried away while the legs are still fresh and push too hard racing the people around you, but it's important to resist this temptation and stick to your own plan from the off. Despite this, we hit the first hill and pumped it out way too hard and I could feel my heart rate rising with the effort. I wasn't happy to be hanging off their coat-tails exhausting myself in the first ten minutes, so I hit the front and brought the tempo down a little. We had to average about 15 miles an hour over the whole course and, keeping this in mind on the first downhill section, I rolled my legs out at a comfortable pace of about 19 miles an hour. No one complained or was pushing to the front, so we held this pace through the first undulating section of the course and on into Pembroke Town. I felt good, the air was fresh and the sun was shining. I was sticking to a liquid-only fuelling plan with about 100 calories every 20 minutes from the watered-down gels in my bottles. I needed to treat this as a genuine Ironman warm-up event, so all the things I was planning to do come race day would have to be practised and refined here.

We were now entering the first hilly section of the course and Muzz, in his typical no-nonsense style, stood up from his saddle and pumped out the steeps like they barely existed, whilst Tom and I clicked quickly through every gear we had till we'd run out and then puffed our way up spinning our legs as fast as we could.

This early part of the course is undoubtedly one of the most beautiful sections, as it makes its way out to the beach at Freshwater West and the headland. We shared the effort and started to overtake a few groups of earlier starters, which made us feel good and encouraged us to keep the effort a little higher than maybe we should have, but we all felt strong and we were riding well, so kept the tempo high as we crested a gentle incline to see the sparkling Atlantic Ocean stretching out in front of us beyond the golden strip of sand and the gently breaking waves at Freshwater West. With the sun on our faces and that view in front of us we were in a good place as we swept down the steep incline along the beach and on into the sand dunes.

We took our time through the dunes as sand had blown on to the road and our skinny tyres wouldn't have taken much encouragement to slide out from underneath us and bring an abrupt and painful end to our race. I made another mental note of this for the big day. Straight through the dunes and we were heading into one of the stiffest climbs of the day to bring us back up from the beach. Again it was click click click back into the highest gear and spinning it out as Muzz charged off into the distance still in his big ring, leaving us to pick our way through wobbling bicycles and people who were already off and pushing on the steepest sections.

Cresting the top, we came back together and were off again and on to the quickest part of the course as we rode back towards Pembroke. This was my chance to prove a bit of fitness and take a decent stint on the front of the group. I had my aero bars fitted and this was the only section where I could really tuck in and take full advantage of them, so I accelerated to the front and got down on them. The aerodynamic effect really does make a difference especially at higher speeds, and I took advantage and slowly increased the pace. Tom and Muzz tucked in behind and we were flying along. I felt great and kept rolling it out. Muzz was sticking to me like glue and taking advantage of the slipstream I was providing but Tom has since told me he was hanging on to the back for dear life and was nearly dropped a couple of times as he struggled to keep up.

As we neared Pembroke we dropped into a long downhill and I began to coast as they both glided past me and tucked in for a speedy descent back into the town. I am not a good descender, I don't really have the nerve to drop down on the bars and let it all go, so by the time I had hit the flat I had to work hard again to catch them back up.

A short steep incline into the town gave me my first hint of the trouble I had to come. As I rounded a sharp uphill corner and hit a steep section, I faded spectacularly. Suddenly, and with no warning, my legs turned to jelly and I wobbled up the hill out of the saddle with my heart rate racing and legs burning as I tried my best to keep up. It took me a long time to recover from that effort and having been on this course before, I knew the hardest parts were still to come. It was definitely my turn to tuck in behind and try to ride out the next few miles to the first of the aid stations.

I insisted we stop as I really needed to get some sugar in me. I used the excuse that I needed to use the toilet to make sure of it, as there was no way they were going to risk riding behind me in that state. I could sense that they were eager to just sail through and were both itching to get going again as we coasted into the aid station. I hadn't told them how rough I was feeling at that point and was hoping that the jelly beans and banana pieces I was stuffing into my mouth and pockets would sort me out quickly enough to not have to. I was already beginning to regret the effort I'd put into that last section, which had clearly run my tank down to pretty much empty.

Straight out from the aid station is a very long draggy uphill. The sun was now beating down on us and I rolled it out as best I could while trying to keep the heart rate down and waiting for the sugar overdose I'd just consumed to start kicking in. It didn't, and what followed was the worst hour on a bicycle I had ever experienced. The course from the aid station is pretty much uphill until the next major town of Narbeth. It was all I could do to grimly keep turning my pedals to keep on the wheel of the person in front. Every gentle incline felt like a mountain and my legs were burning with lactic acid at even the sniff of a hill. My fingers and toes were tingling and I felt sick by the time we'd crested out yet another steep climb into Narbeth town centre. There was a big crowd out to greet us all and I managed to find a little bit of extra energy to style it out down the high street under the bunting, before slumping back over my bars as we rode away from town and into another long incline.

The way I was feeling I knew that this wasn't just a lack of fitness, it was a fuelling problem as I had burnt far too many calories and was bonking badly. Bonking is the term used by cyclists to describe a sudden and alarming lack of energy. My tactic of liquid-only fuelling was clearly not working for me, especially with the spike in effort put in during a competitive event versus training. Added to the exertions in the swim the night before, I had underestimated what I needed and if I did that during the Ironman it would spell the end of my race without a doubt. So I needed to think long and hard about what was required to get it right.

Tom and Muzz were starting to leave me behind and no matter how much I wanted it, I just couldn't keep up. They waited for me at the second aid station and I told them that I'd had it and would need some time out to properly refuel. We were well ahead of schedule, so I was relieved that they were happy to take a break as I found a shady spot to plonk myself down and drink two full bottles of energy drink and eat a flapjack. After a few minutes I was feeling a bit better and the pins and needles in my fingers had gone, so we set off again back towards the coast.

This last section would take us along the coast with the sea to our left at Wiseman's Bridge and Saundersfoot. It is the most dramatic section of the course, with the two steepest climbs coming between the two bays right at the end of the course. This is where the race drama happens and the real test of stamina begins. The climb from Wiseman's Bridge through the woods is the steepest and most sustained climb of the day. I've not had to get off and walk a climb for a long time and this was one of my golden rules of cycling. So as my thighs started to cramp about a third of the way up, I really needed to grit my teeth. I was passing people walking and others who were wobbling wildly across the road. The danger here would be someone falling into me and knocking me off while my feet were still clipped into my pedals.

If I stopped I knew my thighs would turn to rock and I'd have to take time out to stretch and then probably push my bike to the top, and a sudden sense of pride kicked in. I would not be getting off the bike today. I pedalled through it and could feel my right thigh pulsing with cramp as I passed someone leaning over their bars and retching into the bushes at the side of the road. Head down, I rolled on and the cramping eased as I made it to the top and started to freewheel down into the next bay. I stood on my pedals and stretched out my legs as I went.

Tom and Muzz were again waiting for me at the top of the next rise and we rolled together into another big crowd who had gathered in Saundersfoot. The last hill out of Saundersfoot has the steepest section of all as you leave the town and is affectionately known as Heartbreak Hill in Ironman Wales folklore. This is as likely as you are going to get to feeling like a pro cyclist as the crowds here are always the biggest and they close in around you to shout encouragement and get a good view of the pain and drama as people grind their way up the hill.

There was a timed 'King of the Hill' competition over the steepest section and as we approached it I shouted at Muzz to get going. I don't think he really knew what was happening but he leapt out of his saddle and charged full pelt up the hill away from us. There was a commentator who called out his name as he passed the timing chip and the people watching cheered loudly in approval as he sailed off around the corner – they could see he was a contender.

I watched him disappear into the distance and dug in for the last weary uphill mile before we all came back together for the run back into Tenby, which was thankfully mostly downhill. We had one last short sharp climb to go before funnelling into the high street where the crowd was absolutely massive. We rolled in as a team, taking in the applause as we approached the finish line. Muzz raised both hands above his head for a finish line photo opportunity before nearly crashing into the organisers who were waving wildly at him to slow down. My legs nearly buckled as I got off the bike and we took a moment to congratulate each other on a great team ride.

We hobbled through the crowd to collect our medals and then made our way straight to the nearest pub for some well-earned rehydration. I could have sat there in the sun for the rest of the afternoon but there was still the small matter of a half-marathon to run and my legs were completely cooked, so adding a hangover into the mix wasn't going to be the wisest move I could have made.

When we looked up the results we couldn't really believe how well we had done. Taking Muzz's finish time we had come a very respectable 76th out of 437 in a time of four hours and 21 minutes, smashing the five-hour time limit we had set for ourselves. Muzz, despite not even realising why or what he was doing, still managed to finish fifth overall in the King of the Hill competition and that made the beer taste even better.

All I had left to do now was work out how I was going to get my wobbly legs working in time for the run the next morning. Oh well, one thing at a time, another pint won't hurt, will it? It didn't.

The Long Course Weekend – Part 3

IF THE bike leg was a test of my resolve and stamina, then the half-marathon was going to be the event which really put my recovering body to the test as I hadn't run anything like that distance in over three years. I was up to ten miles in training so knew I could get it done, but what sort of state would I be in at the end of it? The course was a tough one, taking in the rolling countryside and coastline of South Pembrokeshire. I knew the course well as I had huffed and puffed my way around it plenty of times on the bike. Some of the climbs were extremely steep and I knew I'd be walking some of it. If I wanted to post a decent time then I would have to spin the legs even faster on the descents and the limited flat bits that were available to me.

Although this was ultimately just a stepping stone on my way to the Ironman, I was still feeling pretty competitive about it. You can't help but be swept up by a little bit of competitive spirit when you have invested so much time to train, and I was prepared to go deep to make this race a personal best and even go under two hours ten minutes. That would be a significant achievement for me considering where I was starting from and a time like that would keep me in contention with Tom, who I was still convinced was going to pull a surprise personal best out of the bag to blow me away.

The good old Welsh weather came in overnight with heavy wind and torrential rain rocking the camper van, but by the morning it had subsided to leave a decidedly chilly start as we walked up to the coaches which would take us to the start line in Pembroke, halfway around the full marathon course.

Pembroke Castle is a foreboding slab of towering Norman stone at the end of the high street and is an impressive congregation point for the half-marathoners. As we walked through the huge entrance archway, the heavens opened and we rushed to take cover under the parapets as cold rain rolled in sheets across the courtyard. You could see your breath it was that cold, so we decided to retreat to a steamed-up coffee shop we had just passed on the high street to grab a hot drink and warm up a bit. We still had 40-odd minutes till the gun, so had plenty of time, and the thought of shivering to death with the rest of the half-naked runners while we waited wasn't appealing.

Just before the start the racers are led out through the castle gates by a drum band in a parade along the high street and up to the start line. Despite the weather there were plenty of locals out to wish us well and clap us on our way. In turn, we could clap and encourage the marathon runners who were passing us on the other side of the road as they made their halfway mark. This all made the start to the day feel quite special, so hats off to the organisers for managing such an encouraging and inspiring spectacle to get us on our way.

The rain stopped and there was even a peek of the sun to warm us up a bit as we bunched together for the start. A countdown from ten was initiated and everyone cheered as the gun went off. We slowly shuffled forwards until we had room to break into a jog and then again into our running stride, and before we knew it we were off. The first part of the course was slightly uphill and on a tight single-track road. With so many people finding their stride it was difficult to get into your own steady pace.

Unsurprisingly, I was feeling very tired and was alarmingly out of breath as we passed the first half mile or so. I was running side by side with Tom at this stage and we laughed and chatted the best we could as we gasped for some breath in the cold air. I kept glancing at my sports watch as I knew the pace I needed to average and I wasn't quite there yet. As the crowds began to disperse slightly, I deliberately lifted the pace and tried to relax into a smoother stride. I could feel Tom accelerate alongside me but after a couple of minutes he said that the pace was a bit too strong for him, so if I wanted to go ahead then I should.

The last thing I needed was a stressful sprint race to the line if it was going to be close between us, so I would have to go now at a pace to get me away and to stay away. I didn't want a game of cat and mouse to develop either so I opened the legs maybe a touch too much and felt him drop away behind me. After a couple of minutes I glanced around and couldn't see him anywhere in the crowd so I eased back a little. I was aware that I was working at a harder intensity than anything I had trained at, so I was going to burn out if I wasn't careful.

Without having to worry about the competition, I relaxed and enjoyed the next half a mile. The legs were loosening up and my breathing had settled. I was now on pace and felt good until a familiar little voice chirped up behind me saying, 'Hello mate, I thought you were going to pick it up a bit?' I looked around and there he was, grinning like a buffoon and looking as fresh as a daisy. I had no real reason to be so competitive with Tom but caught up in the moment I was annoyed and concerned that he was starting to play me and I was falling for it. If I wasn't careful I would frazzle out dancing to his tune and I had visions of watching his fat arse cruise past me in the last couple of miles as he said something like, 'Good effort though mate,' knowing just how much it would wind me up.

I had the time to think as we ran side by side again in silence for a few minutes and I composed myself. I knew what I thought I could do in this race and worrying about the bragging rights back in the office and running myself into an injury was not the way to train for an Ironman. This wasn't anywhere near my A-race and it certainly wasn't the time to get swept up in the euphoria of a foot race with a mate who probably didn't even realise we were racing. It was time to look at the watch again, take a breath and manage the race, not my sweaty shadow who was probably just enjoying the wind-up.

Saying all that, I still couldn't help myself putting in another couple of quick minutes to shake him off. The course was now passing through a patchwork of undulating fields on its way to the coast, where the business end of the race really starts. As we ran towards the halfway mark in the village of Manorbier, there is a very steep downhill section leading to the beach before the first real climb back out of the valley. As I ran down to the beach I let the hill take me and my legs span up into a sprint, my knees and abs were taking quite a pounding and I was uncomfortable by the time I eased up as I passed the beach and dunes before making my way up to the castle.

The ten-kilometre race starts at Manorbier Castle in a similar fashion to the half-marathon in Pembroke, so this time I had the honour returned as I was clapped and encouraged up the hill by the runners waiting to start their race. The encouragement was welcome but was a bit of a double-edged sword to be honest. I could have done with walking a bit on the steepest sections but with so many people cheering me on I felt obliged to make an effort and keep running. My stride shortened along with every breath and my heart rate quickly flew through the roof. By the time I crested the top I was gasping and my legs felt like jelly or lead, or both at the same time if that was even possible. I had to take the next mile nice and easy to recover and slowly I got back on track just in time for another long climb up on to the Ridgeway.

As the name suggests, the Ridgeway is the path of an ancient road which passes along the top of the highest hill line in the area. We would climb up on to the ridge and then along it before descending steeply back down again before tackling the final leg into Tenby and the finish back on the high street. As I hit this climb I started to slow down and was forced into a walk. I swung my arms and yomped, military style, up the winding road to maintain the pace as best I could, but the dip in speed was marked and the fear was creeping back. I found myself constantly looking behind me to see if I could spot Tom coming up through the crowd.

By the time I reached the crossroads at the top I was convinced he was there but I just hadn't spotted him, so I took a moment to properly look all the way down the road behind me. There were colourful runners stretching all the way into the distance but no Tom in sight. I breathed a heavy sigh of relief and started jogging up to the junction which would take a right turn on to the Ridgeway and the return for home.

An old man at the side of road shouted out encouragingly, 'Well done lad, nearly at the top.' He was lying to me, the next two miles were a miserable unending uphill struggle to maintain my race pace on my rapidly lactic-acid-filling legs.

The sharp downhill off the Ridgeway couldn't have come soon enough and was blissfully shaded from the sun, which, despite the wintry conditions we started in, was now blazing down on our backs. I let my legs run out as best I could and was well over race pace when I hit the bottom. This was the moment with about one and a half miles to go that I was sure that Tom was going to come gliding past me with a wave, so despite the pain building in my thighs and weak abs, I held the pace from the descent on to the flat and dug deep.

If I discovered my fighting spirit at the Drogo Ten then that last mile into the outskirts of Tenby was where I discovered that I could make my body do something it really didn't want to. I stubbornly held on to that increase in speed all the way to the finish, I constantly looked at my watch to ensure that I wasn't dipping and when I did, I dug deep and pushed on harder. Every spectator who clapped and encouraged me gave me a massive surge in spirit and the confidence to keep going.

Suddenly I wasn't worried about Tom any more. This was the fastest pace I had ever sustained, let alone at the end of a half-marathon, and I knew he wouldn't be able to live with that. The last little hill into Tenby was short and sharp and I ran up it as best I could. By the time I reached the top I was really struggling for breath and the legs were starting to collapse a little bit underneath me, but I told myself to relax, put my shoulders back and slowly I wound the speed back up. I was nearly there, so now was the time to give it everything I had. I strode through the town feeling like an Olympic athlete and as I rounded the corner to the high street and on to the red carpet, a wall of noise hit me.

Music was pumping and each side of the road was lined with people all clapping and cheering me towards the finish line. The discomfort fell away and I enjoyed my moment in the limelight as I flew across the line. With my hands on my knees I gasped for breath and looked up at the official time – I had finished in two hours, six minutes and 46 seconds. I had smashed my personal best of two hours and 19 minutes by miles, and that was on a flat course. I couldn't believe I was well within the two hours ten minutes I had set for myself and was elated and a little bit sick in my mouth all at the same time.

After collecting a medal and some composure, I looked around at the fantastic crowds while I found a spot to cheer Tom home. I couldn't believe how much support there was for this event and how good it felt performing in front of all these people. I took a moment to let it all sink in. Coming so far since the operation, I could have closed the page on my book at that point right there. I thought about how the real work hadn't even really started yet, about all of the challenges I still had to face and I thought about how it would feel to be on the red carpet of an Ironman.

Then I spotted him thundering down the red carpet to finish in a time of two hours and 19 minutes. He was right after all, he wasn't fit enough for a decent time and I had fallen for all his bluffing and gamesmanship, but you know what? He may not have even realised it but he drove me on that day and in the process I went somewhere deep inside me to a place that I had never been before. I discovered that despite all my physical weakness and mental self-doubt, I could push my body harder and faster than my mind ever thought possible. That was the real prize I won that weekend and was even better than the three wonderful medals I'd received.

The Highs and Lows of the Long Distance Triathlete

AFTER THE successes of the Long Course Weekend, it was time to take stock and regroup before the final big push towards the Ironman start line. Between then and now I had one last big obstacle to jump into and run through in the shape of the Ocean Lava Wales Triathlon. This was a middle-distance event, exactly half the distance of the Ironman, and it was going to be my very first triathlon. Some people competing in triathlons for years would see an event like that as the pinnacle of their achievements, but not me as I was still aiming for one of the hardest endurance events in the world.

I was now entering the key stage of my training and the high-volume sessions were predictably beginning to take their toll on my ailing body. I said to myself right at the start of this whole endeavour that I would need to train through some pain and that now started to become the reality. I was constantly sore, particularly around my left side where that bloody third drain was dragged out of me. I knew at the time that some damage had been done, but months on I was still suffering with painful cramps after exercising and I was often left doubled over before I needed to go to the toilet.

My bowels, although much better, still had a nasty habit of taking me by surprise and on more than one occasion on my way to work, I had to abandon the car on the verge and sprint away stiff-legged into the bushes praying that an innocent dog walker wouldn't stumble across me. I didn't go anywhere without some clean underpants and wet wipes tucked safely in my bag or pockets. This was a real concern for race day. I was truly a man of habit these days and that habit was about 9:30 in the morning after a strong coffee. The impact of a four-in-the-morning start combined with a hearty breakfast could have devastating consequences to my routine, let alone the inside of my tri suit. It was a frightening thought and one I didn't like to dwell on.

I could handle these problems because in a way they were of my making, considering I was the one choosing to put myself through a gruelling training programme. What I was struggling with the most was the dodgy shoulder which was starting to play up on long swims and my old Achilles problems which were now flaring up as a simple consequence of overuse. I could either suck it up and roll the dice regarding an injury or I could do something about it. *Be Iron Fit* talked of having a network of professionals around you to ensure your success and the thought of a nice massage every now and then did sound appealing, so I sorted one out.

I already had a fantastic sports massage therapist available to me whom Maria and I had used many times previously, so I started off by booking in a session every two weeks to loosen up my back and legs and hopefully keep the sciatica at bay. Laura always gives a terrific sports massage but she takes no prisoners whilst seeking out those knots in your muscles. You would have thought that having your butt cheeks massaged by someone other than your wife with relaxing spa music tinkling in the background would be a pleasant experience, but believe me, with Laura's elbows digging into your soft tissue it's an eye-watering one to say the least. A toe-curling hour in her garden retreat would leave me a little tender but always at least an inch taller and definitely ready for another long week of exercise.

With all my training sessions pretty much lasting an hour or more, refining my nutritional needs had become an important piece of the jigsaw. Exhaustion is not your friend, so now was not the time to be using the last few weeks before an Ironman to get beach-body ready and I was replacing all the calories I was burning with gels and energy drinks as I exercised. Fuelling and knowing how your body reacts to it under the stress of constant exercise is the key to a successful race. Gastric problems can derail you because under stress, your body might refuse to absorb any more food and then violently expel what you have managed to consume from either end and sometimes both at the same time.

That's why it's important to train your digestive system as hard as your muscles to allow it to absorb copious quantities of fluid and that magic 100 calories every 20 minutes. Some people prefer liquid only, some would rather eat a cheese and pickle sandwich or a sausage roll – the only way you tell which type you are is to experiment. I knew from the Long Course Weekend that fluid only was not the way for me to go, so I was mixing up energy gels and flapjacks on all my long training sessions. Only having one impromptu visit into the bushes along the canal gave me some confidence that I was getting it about right.

My biggest fear of the whole journey was still the swim; the thought of being dragged from rough seas before I'd even got going was haunting my now frequent nightmares. My less-than-sophisticated training strategy of swimming and more swimming was paying off in its own little way. I knew I could do the half-distance in 45 to 50 minutes, even while being dunked and dragged under the water in race conditions. The questions now were how much stamina did I really have for the latter stages and how much more time would the second lap take? The only way to find out was to do it. Was I prepared for it? I'd always say no, even now. I was very intimidated by the distance but one fine Tuesday evening I took myself off to the lake after work and decided out of the blue that it was going to be the day to get the full distance done and bury the ghost of Mr Bird and his bloody whistle once and for all.

The water was chilly but the sun was warm on my back as I glided away to the first buoy with an energy gel tucked into my sleeve, which I was planning to take in the water after three of the five laps I needed to complete that night. I was the first in the water and by the time I staggered back up the bank, cold, giddy and seasick, I was virtually the last one out. It was as long and tough as expected, but I was in control and had swam two and a half miles in one hour and 48 minutes. I couldn't stop smiling on the drive home; never in my wildest dreams would I ever have imagined myself swimming that sort of distance. All I had to do now was tag on my longest-ever cycle ride and longest-ever run and I'd be finished, easy.

I was starving when I got home and couldn't keep my eyes open by about nine o'clock so went to bed. By my reckoning, that would have equated to about 30 miles into my bike leg so I evidently still had some work to do. I resolved to keep swimming in the lake, and, now that I'd completed the full distance, I would do it every two weeks up till race day.

With only six weeks to go, it was time to make the ultimate sacrifice and give up the alcohol. I timed it impeccably with my sister's wedding so in my final swansong I must have drunk my body weight in champagne, wine and real ale. In the end it probably took until race day to sober up anyway. The new rules I had set were one pint a week and only in a social setting where it would be rude not to. There would be plenty of time for a few celebratory/commiserative beers post-race.

The week before the Ocean Lava we took ourselves off in the camper van to Pembrokeshire for yet more reconnaissance rides of the course and some much-needed sea swimming. I wasn't expecting it but that week tested me more than any other in the entire build-up. The sea swimming was tough, with big swells in cold seas making for some thoroughly miserable swimming and the first swim of the week took the ominous title of the most frightening swim I've ever had the pleasure of enduring. Big swells dragged me backwards and forwards over jagged rocks as huge forests of kelp wrapped themselves around my arms and legs and tried to drag me down into the depths where the largest spider crab I'd ever seen was reaching up towards me like a face-hugger from the movie *Alien*. I cut that swim well short of the violently tossing buoy we were trying to swim towards and doggy paddled for my life back to the beach. I swear it was only my wetsuit that saved me from drowning that day. I was eventually hurled on to the sand by a massive wave where I lay exhausted and broken, feeling every inch like the castaway Robinson Crusoe, if Robinson Crusoe happened to be washed up in a gimp suit.

The cycling proved to be just as emotional. Maria and I rode out on a loop of the Ironman course and the headwind from the coast back to Pembroke was completely standing us up. We could barely move forwards into the wind as we battled around and were knackered by the time we got back, after just a 69-mile ride. This is where it sinks in what a cruel hand the Welsh September weather can play in the race. Any number of factors can contribute to your downfall that just wouldn't be present in a race in a more settled climate – all you can do is train for the worst and hope for the best.

A second ride later in the week turned into a real brute. It was two laps of the hilliest sections, taking in all the big climbs and the long slog up to Narbeth. Each lap was about 42 miles and Maria completed the first with me before peeling off for some retail therapy in Narbeth as I rolled on through for a second lap. It was a hot day and the climbing felt relentless. By the time I had wobbled back up the high street into Narbeth I had completed 84 miles in five hours 35 minutes, at exactly my target time of eight hours for the whole Ironman bike, but I was completely broken. For the first time I had to seriously entertain the thought of not finishing. This was me after 80-odd miles of the 112 I had to do, never mind the swim before and the marathon to follow. I could barely walk back to the campsite as my legs were so cooked. As we sat in the shade of a cafe patio, I sucked up yet another difficult lesson along with my coffee and felt a little crestfallen. Maybe my best wasn't going to be good enough – was it too much too soon after my operation after all?

The second week was easier going, as I gave myself a break and tapered down before my initiation into the world of triathlon. The night before the race we drove down to get familiar with the transition area and to take a look at the course. The race was a hilly one but that was exactly what I needed to replicate the conditions of the Ironman. We parked up and looked out at the swim course, which was in the harbour at Fishguard. The water was cold, still and grey. It looked deep, dark and intimidating. Maria was doing the shorter sprint race, so would complete one loop of the swim, whereas

I would need to do an Australian exit from the water, run back to the start ramp about 50 metres away and go back again for a second lap. The cut-off was again one hour, which was still playing on my mind. I was horrified by the thought of not making the transition and being forced to stop.

Race morning came and the buzz was palpable as we checked in for our race numbers and went to rack our bikes. This was the first time that I needed to lay out my kit for transitions and I took the time to organise everything so that I could smoothly go from one discipline into the next. The last thing I wanted was to misplace something and waste time looking for it in an exhausted panic.

It was an early start and before we knew it we were huddled at the start in our wetsuits with around 350 other competitors and lots of supporters all listening to the race briefing. The roads were not closed for the race so attention to traffic and obeying road law was paramount. There was a point on the course which required a complete stop at a T-junction and it was a straight disqualification if the race umpire did not see you put a foot down. The race director asked whose first triathlon it was and I raised my hand with about a third of the field, most of whom were doing the sprint distance. He got everyone to give us a round of applause and congratulated us on breaking our triathlon virginity, which was a nice touch. With one last cheer we all turned around and shuffled to the slipway, which led down to the water's edge.

The nerves were kicking in now but it felt good. I believed I could make the swim cut and just needed to concentrate on maintaining my swim pace right from the start. I turned to Maria and was surprised to see she was crying. 'I'm fine,' she blubbered through the tears, 'I'm just so proud of you for getting here.' I was a little taken aback as I had been concentrating so hard on getting my head right for the start, I didn't appreciate just how significant a moment it was. I gave her a tight squeeze and quickly pulled down my goggles as I appeared to be getting something in my eye as well. She was right, last August when I was diagnosed we had no idea what the future was going to bring and within a year it had brought me here, about to complete one of the toughest triathlons going. Just as we were both about to lose it completely, we were saved by the start gun suddenly going off and with a puff of the cheeks I shuffled forward into the cold, still water of the harbour. My first triathlon had begun.

The concrete slipway angled gently into the water as we all edged forwards. It was a shock to the system when we reached our thighs and the ground suddenly ran out, plunging us straight in. I'd experienced a mass start and knew how difficult it was to get your legs up behind you to swim when people are grabbing you from behind and trying to kick your teeth out in front, so this time I positioned myself right on the edge of the pack. I was able to swim pretty much unhindered from the off, but was already starting to worry as halfway to the first buoy it felt like literally everybody was overtaking me.

'Do not panic,' I said to myself whilst I panicked, 'just relax and swim, you've got this.' Rounding the first buoy the deeper water became freezing cold, still and heavy. It felt like swimming in soup and I was now pretty much on my own. I rounded the second buoy and tried to sight the exit slipway. It was tiny and looked miles away but I managed to block out the thoughts of the deep, dark water beneath me and swam steadily towards it. My hands eventually touched the concrete of the slipway and I rose smoothly out of the water and began jogging back to the start. I looked towards the transition area as I passed it and it seemed that virtually every other competitor was long gone on their bikes or were just about to be; I glanced behind me and took some comfort in the fact that there were still a few heads bobbing in the water.

For the first time in my life I dived head first back into the water to start my second lap. Feeling like a pro, albeit a lonely and very slow one, I headed back out on my second lap. I had no idea what the time was and the last leg back to the exit seemed to be taking forever. The fear was rising now as the steady stream of people getting out ahead of me had turned to a trickle. 'Please let me finish within the cut-off,' I pleaded to myself as I wobbled up the ramp and ran towards a now alarmingly empty transition area. People were cheering and congratulating me and I wasn't being pulled to one side by anyone in a fluorescent vest, so I kept going and sneaked back into the transition area. A quick look at my watch told me I'd finished in 49 minutes and there were still about 50 people left in the water behind me.

As I stripped off my wetsuit I realised how cold I was. My hands were numb and I fumbled as I pulled on my socks and cycling shoes. I blew on my hands to warm them up as I rolled out of the transition area and on to the open roads of Pembrokeshire. I needn't have worried about the cold, as the route took a quick turn uphill and I was soon sweating with the effort as I tried to get some rhythm going. I was tired and realised for the first time the amount of energy that combining events takes out of you. Head down, I plugged away, thinking there was only 56 miles of this to go.

Some of the sprint race cyclists were already flying back down the hill to start their run and I was feeling a little envious seeing them freewheeling past me. Out of nowhere I heard a loud screeching and looked up to see Maria whizzing past cheering and waving wildly. She was clearly relieved that I hadn't drowned and had made the cut-off, and it made me smile and gave me the boost I needed to press on. It was a lonely place out on the course. As a misty rain started to roll across the headland, most of the middle-distance triathletes were long gone up the road and I was locked into a race with the few backmarkers around me. I always had someone to chase up the road though and I triumphantly passed one person before realising he wasn't even in the race and was just out for a leisurely ride in the countryside.

As I reached the beautiful city of St David's, I came up to the foot-down T-junction that was mentioned in the safety briefing. I pulled up to a stop and got a whole lot more than a foot down as inextricably, for the first time in years, my foot got stuck in my cleat and as I desperately tried to unclip I felt myself toppling over sideways in gloriously high-definition slow motion. First in contact with the tarmac with a loud crack was my elbow, followed swiftly by the thud of my helmet and then my knee. I lay on the wet road in shock for a few seconds as a fluorescent-clad volunteer came running to my aid. What an idiot, as if things weren't already hard enough.

As I untangled myself from my bike and staggered to my feet, my elbow was stinging painfully and I could see a big flap of skin hanging down as blood mixed with the rain was freely running down my forearm and into my glove. My kneecap was sore but I seemed to have escaped with nothing more serious than a painful bit of embarrassment. I got back on the bike, which was fortunately also unscathed, and with the help of the concerned volunteer I pedalled away as fast as I could from the small crowd that was now gawping at me with open mouths from under their umbrellas.

Out of town and back on the open road, I could focus again and see about reining a few people in. I tucked into my aero bars and winced as the cut on my arm stuck to the foam elbow pad and reopened itself. The rain had now stopped and the sun appeared for the first time that day. It felt good and the remainder of the bike leg was far less dramatic, but the biggest issue I now faced was the local roads themselves that had been freshly redressed with loose gravel just in time for 300 pairs of skinny wheels to roll over them. It forced me to take a lot of speed off, especially on the twisty descents. A nasty crash on that surface would have taken the skin from more than my elbow, that was for sure, and I didn't fancy riding back into transition half-naked with a bloodstained arse cheek hanging out of a shredded tri suit.

I managed to overtake about a dozen people on the run in and nobody came past me, which felt good. When I finally got my chance to roll down that steep descent back into the transition I was pleased how the race was going. I was back into transition exactly where I thought I'd be, at around four hours and 20 minutes.

I pulled on my trainers and the obligatory triathlete's sun visor – if nothing else I did look the part as I thrust a banana down my throat and trotted back out on to the run course. There were a lot more people around now, with runners all over the course at different stages of their races. The course was four laps, each consisting of a soul-destroying and energy-sapping long flat section into a headwind along the harbour wall to the lighthouse and then back across the fields along the shoreline, before rising steeply on to the clifftop footpath which itself then rose up sharply. Some comedian had written SORRY! in chalk across the path at one particularly steep section and this comedy genius was only outdone by the REALLY SORRY! greeting you just before the near-vertical section at the highest point of the course. It was here that you stretched out a weary arm and were presented with a coloured arm band by the smiling volunteers to signify the completion of each lap. From there it was all downhill as you weaved through a housing estate passing an old grandma who, bless her, had sat on her front lawn the whole day cheering, and then back to the harbour where you would turn around and do it all again.

I was alarmed at how leaden my legs were as I tried to roll myself up to speed out of the transition – it was clear now that the cumulative exhaustion of a triathlon can only be replicated by doing a triathlon and it wasn't a pleasant sensation. Legs that have just spent three or more hours spinning one way just don't want to start spinning in another as you begin to run. After a few minutes of hobbling and hopping I finally found a pace, but it wasn't a comfortable one. I gritted my teeth and let the distraction of the crowds take my mind off it. Maria kept mine and several others' spirits up by leaping like a gnome from the bushes at random points around the course and cheering us on in her big purple bobble hat.

As each lap dragged by, I was begging for the uphill sections to come again just so I'd have an excuse to walk for a bit. You learn another important lesson at this stage of a race, that it really is mind over matter. You may not be able to bang out a massive extra effort but the concentration required to even start running again and then maintain a pace, despite the pain, is all-consuming. The desire to stop is sometimes overwhelming but you know the pay-off you are working towards, so you must find a way to distract yourself and carry on. I tried my best and despite nearly vomiting on the most hideously textured vanilla energy gel I have ever tasted, twice, I eventually made it back on to the flat and the last kilometre into the finishing straight.

This was the time to really give whatever was left in the tank. My legs were like solid blocks of wood and had been on the verge of cramping for the last hour, but I rolled them out of a jog and into a run as the red carpet and the finishing arch came ever closer. The finish was glorious. There may have only been Maria plus one man and his dog left to greet me when I eventually got there, but nothing could take away how good it felt to run down that red carpet and up the ramp on to the stage to collect my medal as the announcer called out my name over the loudspeakers.

Sat on the harbour wall a few minutes later nursing a bottle of water and looking at the impressive chunk of metal hanging around my neck, I couldn't believe it. I'd completed a middle-distance triathlon in six hours and 47 minutes. My run time of two hours and 25 minutes, although not quick, was only six minutes slower than my previous best half-marathon on the flat all those years back. I had indeed come a long way. I felt lean and fit but fuck me, halfway? Really?

There was still a lot of work to do, but following the lows of the week before this was a high and a bloody big one. I was going to enjoy the moment for now and worry about the small matter of that other race another day.

The Final Push

TWO DAYS after the Ocean Lava I was back at the lake to resume my training. I didn't want to take time off as any rest period I treated myself to would only have dragged on to at least the end of the following week. I figured I was better off getting straight back on the horse. I was off work in good time, and as I was changing into my wetsuit at the lake in the sunshine I made the decision to make it a five-lap, two-and-a-half-mile kind of day, seeing as I was now a bona fide triathlete.

The water was surprisingly chilly as I slid in and lifted my feet to dunk my head. It rolled down my back into my wetsuit and made me shiver, but I soon warmed up as I began swimming the now familiar route out towards the first buoy. I swam purposefully but not fast, as I knew I had to preserve something for later, and along the back of the lake I watched the fish swimming below me and the ducks in the shallows and I felt pretty good, but by the end of the second lap I was starting to feel the effects of the weekend's efforts. I kept my head down and looked away from the exit point as I passed it to avoid the temptation to swim straight towards it and get out.

As the swim went on I could feel my strength slowly ebbing away; my stroke, which isn't great at best, had become ragged. My arms were flapping at the water and my legs were being dragged uselessly behind me. As I finished the third lap I realised how cold I was becoming and again it took all my willpower to swim past the jetty as a stream of people were already sensibly climbing out and going home.

It had clouded over at some point during that last lap and without the sun on my back I was physically starting to shiver. I tried my best to speed up and warm up, but the harder I tried the slower I got. I simply did not have it in me. I didn't realise how much the triathlon had taken out of me and I was completely spent as I willed myself to keep going on to that fifth lap.

I knew it was a bad move as I rounded the first buoy with about 700 metres to go. Up until then I had been sharing the water with other swimmers but as it started to get dark I was the only person I could see left in the leaden water. I knew it was a painfully slow swim and when I finally dragged myself from the water, the watch told me I had taken over two hours to get it done. I felt sick, giddy and was shivering uncontrollably – the effort it had taken had been massive.

When I eventually got home and told Maria, she was annoyed, saying that I shouldn't have even been attempting such a big swim so soon after the Ocean Lava. She was right, all I had succeeded in doing was bringing back the spectre of a timeout on the Ironman swim, but after some dinner and a warm shower I finally stopped shivering and started to feel a bit more positive. I reflected that it had actually been good mental training if nothing else. No physical damage was done and I had proved to myself that when the going got tough I was able to focus and get through it. Despite my worst swim in months, I still completed more than the full distance and was still within the cut-off. I decided to take the positives and those few days off after all.

By the end of the week I was back on it and some of my longest training sessions were now coming thick and fast. I was running half-marathons and cycling 80-odd miles in a single weekend, which was crazy considering that only a year before a half-marathon was the absolute pinnacle of my achievement.

All this exercise was now starting to break me down as much as it built me up though, and for a few weeks my Achilles problems had started to niggle me. After a hilly ten kilometres one evening, I found myself limping painfully after my shower. The next day I was still walking around on tiptoes and was seriously worried about the escalation in the pain and stiffness I was experiencing. Both Achilles were literally creaking as I walked and they were painful to touch. I was now only a month out from the race and this was when the most important long sessions were kicking in. As it was, I was only doing the 'Just Finish' programme and I really couldn't afford to miss any training at this stage.

As I phoned around for an urgent physiotherapy appointment, the doubts about my ability were once again roaring around inside my head. I had been so focussed on my training that I had managed to push these thoughts away when I was happily hitting my milestones. The blessing of knowing the race course so well was also coming back to bite me as I went over everything that could go wrong.

What didn't figure much in my thoughts was the cancer. My body in some ways wasn't what it was before the operation. I was physically very fragile, but in many ways I was in so much better shape – I had dropped a lot of weight and was certainly much fitter and stronger. My focus was fully on racing and any thoughts about recurrences and complications had been well and truly buried for now.

I got an urgent physiotherapy appointment and after a quick examination my therapist, Kelly, could see that my calves were incredibly tight and there was a mass of scarring on both my Achilles tendons. She couldn't cure it before the race but the good news was that we could treat it and maintain it to allow me to continue training and compete. I was delighted to hear this but wasn't as delighted when she started to get to work. As she pressed her thumbs through my calves and Achilles tendons I could feel balls of tension tearing and loosening. As I lay face down on her table sweating, a little tear rolled down my cheek. This was almost as bad as my time in hospital. I told myself it was for the best and it certainly proved to be just that.

I walked out of the clinic and back to the car on wobbly legs but already felt like I could straighten up and stretch out my Achilles painlessly. My role in my recovery was to heat my Achilles each night to encourage blood flow and then come back each week for more of the same. A few days later I was back running more freely and my confidence started returning with every pain-free session I completed.

One of my last training rides was another of those exercises in just finishing as I ground my way around a hilly 40-mile circuit in the pouring rain. It was cold and miserable and the farmer's track I found myself cycling down, looking for a short cut home, had left me splattered in cow shit and wet clay. As I rolled back on to smooth tarmac, I could feel my back wheel wobbling alarmingly and looked down to see I had a puncture. I pulled over to the verge and, running my numb fingers around the rim to find the hole, I sliced my thumb open on what looked like a Neolithic arrow head sticking out of my back tyre. The rain and blood was running down my arms and pouring off my fingers as I leant forward. Filthy dirty and cursing loudly, I fumbled around fitting a new inner tube whilst slowly developing hypothermia.

I managed to swim the full distance once more in those last couple of weeks and finished comfortably at one hour 47 minutes – I had only gone and done it. Up yours Bird! With your too-tight shorts, mushroom floats and little faith, I was an Ironman distance swimmer after all.

With two weeks to go, the hard work was done and I was now tapering down. This is traditionally the time when athletes say they feel at their weakest, most injured, emotional and unsure of themselves. They call it the taper blues, and even though I had missed virtually none of my last sessions I was not escaping the feelings, and with one week to go I went and tweaked my shoulder on my last swim. This was the injury I feared the most of all. I couldn't believe after months of training with no problems it was coming back to haunt me right now. All I could do was take some painkillers, rest and hope for the best.

As I now had some spare time on my hands, I could sit back and look at the raft of training data I had collected and make a realistic assessment of my chances. I calculated the swim would take one hour 45, the bike leg a full eight hours and the marathon, five hours on a good day.

These were what I considered to be good times that would get me around in 15-odd hours, two hours before the cut-off. The critical section for me was the bike leg. I knew that I would be taking eight hours to complete those 112 miles and this would only leave me with about 45 minutes before the bike cut-off. This was the tightest section of the whole race and with that much distance to cover anything could happen – two punctures or a mechanical failure would bring me way too close for comfort and who knew what a crash might take out of me? This is where the biggest prospect of failure was – to be precise, it was just 24 seconds a mile that was the difference between my success and failure.

The bike was packed off to the local shop for a full service and I also fitted new inner tubes and new tyres with some time to bed them in. I had all my kit laid out in piles around the spare bedroom and checked off my kit lists over and over to make sure I didn't forget anything. It was all starting to get very real.

With just a couple of days to go, my shoulder relaxed but I developed another bout of painful sciatica in my right buttock and down the back of my leg. Bloody hell what next, was I just being a hypochondriac or was I genuinely starting to fall apart?

My sports massage therapist, Laura, let me borrow an electric massager to use in the lead-up to the race. It looked like a frightening medieval torture device crossed with something you might buy from the Ann Summers website, but it seemed to do the trick. Maria took great delight in leaning her full weight on it as it pummelled my arse cheeks and my sciatica into submission.

That last week dragged by slowly; all I had thought about for the last year was that bloody race, and it couldn't come quick enough. The all-consuming nature of it was now starting to wear me down. I had trained as best as I could, I hadn't cut any corners and I knew my pace was good enough to get me around if I could keep going for that length of time and avoid any serious incidents. The longest sustained single session I had performed was still the Wales Triathlon and I finished that absolutely spent. I hoped that this was partly down to the psychology of crossing the finishing line and a bit of a mental re-adjustment would keep me going past that seven-hour mark.

I had booked a bed and breakfast in Tenby town centre for us as soon as I had booked the race, and we were in a prime town-centre location right next to the transition area and finish line. The owners had reserved the whole property for competitors and their families on race weekend and it took a lot of pressure off knowing that we were well sorted up front, with no travelling to do.

Parking was a problem on such a busy weekend but this was sorted well in advance as well. We had packed up the camper van to drive down and I had booked it into a local campsite so my best mate Luigi and his son could camp in it.

Along with Tom and myself, Tom's brother Paul, his wife Gwen and Tom's friend Graham were also taking part. They were all staying within walking distance in caravans and we had a chance to meet up on the Friday evening over a barbecue. I avoided the prawns, not wanting to take any unnecessary risks just two days before the event, and it was great to meet up with everybody and have a good laugh to take away some of the tension.

Earlier that day we had walked into town to the exposition area where I could collect my Ironman rucksack with my numbers, swim cap and timing chip inside. Passing through the tent, all the Ironman merchandise was laid out and looked great. People were buying it up in their droves, but there was no way I was going to tempt fate and waste my money buying random Ironman-branded tat until the Monday morning when I had that medal hanging around my neck. My tea would taste pretty bitter from an Ironman Wales mug if I didn't even finish.

In the afternoon we had to go to a nearby airfield for the race briefing. There were hundreds of athletes and their families crowded into a large hangar and the compère started whipping up the atmosphere. The infectious excitement being generated made us feel like we were about to undertake something very special. Tom said that he could tell who all the serious athletes were as they were the ones always sitting down to preserve their energy, but it looked to me like everyone was sitting down to be honest and more than a few appeared to be just plain exhausted, injured or both.

When all the athletes were together like this it showed just how many people appeared to be carrying injuries – there were a lot of taped limbs on show and I was grateful that all I had to contend with was a numb arse cheek; all things can be put into some sort of perspective.

The following morning I gave the bike one last check over and filled my transition bags with my bike and running kit. Now was not the time to forget something, so the checklists were out and all the items were counted in one at a time, including all the nutrition and chamois cream for my sensitive sweaty bits. When I was finally happy, I tipped it all out and packed it again for good measure. Finally content that I had everything, I shouldered my bags and wheeled my bike through the gates into a huge bike-racking area. My race number was 1463 and I found my spot in the racking and propped up my bike, I took one last look over it, to be sure, and with a tap on the saddle I told him to rest up and I would see him in the morning.

I knew that it was going to be a tough day out and I was going to need all the help I could get, so perusing the internet for some more essential rubbish to buy I saw some personalised stickers for your bike's crossbar. I had a think about what profound prose I could look down at during the tough times to help me get going again. It was no contest, I knew exactly what I was going to have on my sticker.

'GET A GRIP, this isn't drain 3 being removed!'

If I needed a more miserable, painful life moment to reflect back on then that was it. Nothing I would experience in the race could touch that and if I could remind myself of this when I was feeling weak and sorry for myself, then it should give me the kick up the arse I would undoubtedly need at some point.

As we walked back to the hotel we passed by the finish line, which the staff were busy readying for the IronKids race that evening. I stood at the bottom of the long red carpet stretching out in front of me and, looking at the finishing arch in the distance, I made a quiet promise to be seeing that view tomorrow evening even if it killed me. Maria wanted me to step on to the red carpet for a photograph but I declined. The first steps I took on that magical carpet would be when I was just about to become an Ironman and not a second before.

Tom's daughter was doing the IronKids event so we all congregated on the small grandstand erected at the finishing straight to cheer her through. There was a big crowd clapping the kids in and the atmosphere was great. As I stood there, so close to the finish line with the music pumping and the sheer joy of everyone applauding and having a good time, I looked up at the Ironman Wales logo and suddenly started to well up.

Before I knew it the tears were streaming down my cheeks as the emotion of a whole year suddenly poured out of me. Just being there at that finish line meant so much when I didn't even know if I would be alive to see it. Everything I had gone through during the operation and afterwards and the sacrifices we had all made to get here washed over me and I couldn't control it. I turned away from my family and wiped my face – I was a bit embarrassed as I'm definitely not one for public shows like this. I could see a couple of people had noticed me and were wondering if I was alright. I was definitely alright; in fact, I was delighted, and those tears soon turned to emotional laughter. I was determined to enjoy every moment of this journey and right there and then nothing was going to stop me.

After the IronKids we said our goodbyes and went for an early dinner back in the room. I didn't want to take any chances again so we took the rice cooker with us and enjoyed a meal of plain rice and cooked chicken breast with a tin of kidney beans and a chicken stock cube stirred into it. We watched a bit of television and then set and checked every available alarm clock in the room. I applied my race number tattoos and it was time for an early night.

It goes without saying that I didn't sleep a wink, and after six restless hours staring at the ceiling in a darkened hotel room, with Maria tossing and turning in the bed next to me, all the alarm clocks went off in unison. It was ten past four in the morning.

Finally, after a very long year, it had arrived. It was race day.

Swim

I TURNED the light on, got straight out of bed and started fumbling with our phones to stop the alarms disturbing anybody else. I needn't have worried as I could hear at least another two going off in the rooms around us. Maria squinted out from under the duvet and her wild bed hair, 'Euurrrgghh, I'm knackered, how are you feeling?'

I felt surprisingly awake and focussed, despite the early hour. The first thing I noticed as I walked around the room was that the sciatica which had plagued me for the last few days seemed to have disappeared and my shoulder also felt fine. I miraculously appeared to have made it to race morning uninjured.

My clothes and my race chip were piled neatly on the chair and as I dressed I pulled on my calf guards, which I was planning to wear for the duration of the race. The jury was still out on the benefit they had provided me in training, but I had worn them throughout and my perception was that they controlled my calf muscles and hence my fragile Achilles heels, so I wasn't going to break the habit now.

The hotel was all geared up for breakfast from 4am, so after a quick cup of tea in the room we headed down. My routine was well prepared and I had with me my tin of rice pudding. The whole tin was going to be the basis of my breakfast, along with some strong coffee to hopefully get the bowels moving at that ungodly hour, all to be washed down with about one litre of tropical-flavoured isotonic energy drink. The landlady warmed my rice pudding for me and I stirred in a spoonful of honey and jam for a bit of extra energy.

There were three other athletes in the breakfast room all looking apprehensive; we wished each other luck and shared some nervous jokes. One of the guys said it was his fifth Ironman Wales. He had completed them all since it started – hats off to the effort that he must take to train to that intensity each year. Unbelievable, knowing what it took to get me to the start.

After breakfast I was back up in the room pulling on my tri suit and wetsuit whilst belching rice pudding and trying not to be sick in my mouth every time I bent down. I was busy dressing because I'd already spent far too long sat on the toilet trying not to strain as I waited for the inevitable not to happen. I was concerned because, with my delicate digestive tract, this first failure to perform was going to cause me some problems later in the day, but there was nothing I could do about it now. Some people suggest dosing up on Imodium to avoid any gastric issues, but I figured that if I did that, I could be making matters worse and would just give myself hideous cramps to contend with. If it came down to it, I would have to find a bush out on the course somewhere.

All I had left to do now was put my bottles and energy drinks on to the bike and make my way down to the beach and prepare for the start. It was really happening. I was surprisingly calm still but I could now feel some apprehension beginning to rise in me, despite the fact that I knew there was no point fretting at this late stage; whatever was going to come my way today was going to happen whether I liked it or not. In the transition area and alone with my thoughts, I took a few deep breaths as I fitted my bottles to the bike and put some gels and flapjacks into the pouch on my crossbar. The earliest of dawn's light was just starting to peek over the horizon and it cast a soft glow over the rows and rows of bikes racked silently together. There was a hushed urgency in the air as athletes made their own final personal preparations around me.

It's surprising how many loud bangs you hear coming out of the gloom in the transition area as people over-inflate their tyres. What an absolute nightmare trying to change an inner tube or, even worse, sourcing a new tyre with only an hour before the whistle. I couldn't think of a worse start to the day. I squeezed my own tyres and they felt good and firm as I had inflated them the night before; my bike was ready to go and so was I. Taking one last look at the motivational sticker on the crossbar, I smiled – let's see just how painful this race can be, then. If it is going to be worse than drain three then I was in big trouble.

I made my way out of the transition to where Maria was waiting and we walked together through the dense crowds down towards the harbour. There were big crowds out to see the race and it made me feel proud to be part of the spectacle they were all there to witness. You couldn't be mistaken for anything other than a competitor as you marched around in your wetsuit with a face looking like a slapped arse.

As we neared the north beach we met up with Tom, his brother Paul, Paul's wife Gwen and Tom's friend Graham. We had been foolish enough to sign up all those months back and had all managed to make it to the start in one piece. As we lined up for one last photo before we went down, I looked at each of them and hoped that we could all get to that finish line and be photographed with our medals. That thought gave me an extra nugget of motivation to ensure I held up my side of that bargain.

Some people prefer to fly below the radar on an event like this for fear of failure, but I didn't feel the need for that. First and foremost, this race was for me, but I didn't shy away when it came to letting people know what I was up to. I figured that the pressure I would put on myself to finish was more than enough, so the expectation of others was not a bigger burden to carry – if anything it would help spur me on.

I was of course fearful of failure, but if it happened I didn't feel that I would be letting myself or anybody else down considering what I had gone through. A lot of friends had come down to cheer me on and a whole lot more were going to monitor my progress through their computer screens throughout the day. I had told myself all year that making the start line was the real achievement, but now I was standing here, that was clearly a load of bollocks. I really wanted that medal.

We made our way to the beach and as we got nearer the athletes were funnelled off from the crowds behind barriers so that they could get down to the beach unhindered. I said my goodbyes to Maria and she told me how proud she was and that she loved me. I saw another tear in her eye as we embraced one last time. I told her I would see her at the finish line and turned to make my way down through the crowds to the start. I had about 20 minutes to get myself together.

As the transition from the swim to the bikes is over one kilometre long with a steep zigzag path to negotiate, you get an extra transition bag to put some trainers in and to carry your wetsuit if you decide to take it off. I had a bottle of water to squirt the sand off my feet and a banana in mine, in addition to my old trainers. Walking down the zigzag, there were row upon row of these purple bags hanging on racking and as I found my spot and hung my bag, I made a mental note of where I had put it so I could go straight to it when I came out of the water. The previous year I had seen some hapless, clearly exhausted unfortunates running up and down the line in a panic looking for their bags, so I wanted to make sure I wasn't one of them.

This was the first year that the Ironman organisation was trialling a rolling-swim start, so instead of everybody crowding on the beach together, as we had witnessed the previous year, we were now queued in an orderly fashion along the sea wall back towards the harbour. There were timing markers to allow us to get into groups of similar ability. I seemed a long way back down the line at one hour 45 but there were still at least 200-odd people behind me.

Tom had wandered forwards looking for the sign that said 'Vikings' as a stranger helped me pull the zip up on the back of my wetsuit. I pulled on my red Ironman swim cap and goggles and pressed them tightly on my cheeks, feeling the suction as they sealed to my face. I was worried about them leaking and getting an eyeful of salty water. I'd heard horror stories of people losing their goggles completely and having to finish the sea swim without them, not something I wanted to contemplate. My goggles were pretty much brand new for the race and felt good. I hitched them back up and looked around. There was some hushed but excitable chatter as the dawn started giving way to the morning and the bay was beginning to be lit up by milky sunlight.

We were all patting each other on the back and wishing each other the best of luck. There were no real feelings of competition this far down the pack, just a determination and a desire for all of us to have a good race and get the job done. Looking out into the bay, the sea looked pretty calm. I was happy with the conditions and was quietly confident I had it within me to get the swim done.

Out of the blue I heard the stirring strains of the Welsh anthem, 'Land of My Fathers', drifting across the bay. I could hear people around the clifftops singing and I blew out my cheeks and took a few deep breaths as goose bumps erupted all over me. I felt tears coming again as it really sunk in that I was here, and despite everything I had endured to get there I was about to show myself and the cancer that I was strong enough to overcome it.

I heard the horn sound for the start and there were loud cheers from the galleries and adrenaline-filled whoops from the athletes around me as tensions were released and we slowly started to shuffle forwards to the start line on the beach. I wiped my eyes, pulled down and reset my goggles and put on my nose plug. I had a second plug on my finger like a ring and an inhaler and an energy gel tucked up my wetsuit sleeves – I was completely ready to go.

The crowd of athletes slowly started to move faster and faster as we approached the start, but it still took a full seven minutes for me to be greeted by the crescendo of beeps as timing chips activated around me and at last we stepped down on to the sand to begin our races. Suddenly there was space around me and I got a direct look at the sea and the first buoy bobbing in the distance. The water was alive with thrashing arms and red swim caps for as far as I could see, and it was a fantastic sight to behold from the water's edge as I jogged easily down the beach and into the water.

The water was cold on my feet but nothing I wasn't used to. There were a few small waves lapping the beach but it looked as calm as I had imagined as I started to wade out to my waist. I must have drunk about two litres of fluid already that morning and now was the time to let it all go before I started swimming. I flooded my wetsuit with a gloriously warm glow and ploughed out into the deeper water. I was now up to my chest and people around me had started to swim. I kept walking until I was up to my shoulders and once again I had to physically tell myself to start bloody swimming. I dived forwards and under the water and felt the cold sea rush into my wetsuit and down my back. I came up, took a deep breath and kicked with my feet to bring them up behind me and take my first strokes out into the bay.

I wasn't a quick swimmer and I knew from my experiences in the lake and pool that the more I thrashed around the slower I got. I knew exactly what my rhythm was and I needed to get into it and stick to it. As I swam I sighted the first buoy and planned to swim as directly as I could towards it. I couldn't afford to swim miles out of my way or zigzag wildly around the course. I could already see other swimmers fanning out a long way from the pack, but it was absolutely critical for my time to know where I was in the water at all times and swim in a straight line. I found myself laughing as I swam. I felt great and couldn't believe I was actually doing it; fuck me, I was really swimming 2.4 miles in the sea during an actual Ironman. It was crazy and my feelings of apprehension were now melting away into excitement and maybe a little bit of hysteria, if I'm honest.

My happy thoughts were soon rudely interrupted as a huge arm loomed up from my left and came crashing down on to my head. I didn't see it coming and it hit me just as I was turning away to take a breath. My head was dunked just as I breathed in and I was suddenly sucking a huge mouthful of salty water into my lungs. I spluttered for breath and tried to regain some composure as a giant walrus of a man started to swim across me, this time clouting me painfully across the back with the same heavy-trailing arm. My legs sunk under me and I looked around to see what exactly had just come over the top of me. It felt like I had been hit by a boat.

In an instant my smile was gone and my race face was suddenly well and truly on. I consider myself to be a considerate chap and I work hard to ensure I keep out of other people's way in a swim. This fucker clearly couldn't have given a shit and the red mist descended quickly once I'd got my breath back. He was still swimming diagonally across me so as he got up alongside me again I gave him a good downwards and outwards shove in the back as hard as I could to simultaneously push him away and dunk him under. He was clearly about as accomplished a swimmer as I was as he rolled almost fully on to his back and his arms started flailing as he tried to keep his head above the water. He spluttered away to my left and I dove down into the water to bring my legs back up behind me and get away from him; fortunately, that was the last I saw of that idiot.

I was nearing the first buoy now and could feel the swell of the ocean rising as I was much further out into the bay. The water was raising me up and dropping me down with each stroke and I could see a familiar scrum of swimmers stuck in a crowd at the first buoy, so I took the decision to go wide, having learned the lesson from the Long Course Weekend. I swam around the bobbing heads and back into clear water beyond the buoy and out into the deep grey water of the bay.

I saw the second buoy in the distance by the harbour wall. This was a long drag through the fishing boats and diesel spills parallel to the beach, and here it was even more crucial to swim in a straight line and not waste any time or energy swimming off course. The swell was massive and so much bigger than it had appeared from the beach, great big rolling waves were swinging across the bay in front of me. At times I was plunging down into the troughs of the waves and at others I found my arms flailing in the air as I tried to swim over the top of them. It was harder swimming than I was used to but I still felt strong, so I ploughed forwards as best I could.

The clouds of jellyfish were huge out in the bay, and every time my face was in the water I could see dozens of tiny opaque creatures whizzing past my goggles. Just as I was thinking how beautiful they looked, I felt a sharp sting across my lip and up across my right cheek where a trailing tentacle had brushed across my face. I felt it stick and pull at my lip and cheek before just as quickly detaching itself and moving away. The burning pain was instant and sharp. I rolled on to my back and frantically rubbed my face; for fuck's sake, if this day wasn't going to be hard enough I now had to contend with this. I rolled back on to my front and got going again. The cold water was probably numbing the sting but I could feel my lip and cheek swelling by the minute.

As I rounded the second buoy I could see and hear people calling out encouragement from the harbour wall. It's a lonely place when you are head down in the water and the presence of some support close by makes you realise you are still actually in a race and was very welcome. I felt the presence of a few swimmers speeding past me as I turned for the beach and the end of my first lap. These must have been the elite athletes who would shortly be finishing their swims; I, on the other hand, had been in the water for about 40 minutes and still had another hour to go.

I swam for the beach and I could see the crowds on the clifftops. Each time my head lifted from the water I could hear the music pumping in the distance. I could see the Ironman banners and the inflatable transition arch marking the end of the swim. As usual, every time I looked up it just didn't seem to be getting any closer no matter how far I swam. It wasn't the time to panic though. Everything had gone to plan despite the jellyfish sting, which now felt like an alarmingly throbbing trout pout. 'Just swim to your rhythm and you will get there,' I told myself. Eventually my hands touched the sand and I rose shakily to my feet and started to jog up the beach to the timing mat and the turn back towards the sea.

I pulled the energy gel from my sleeve and tore off the top with my teeth. As I jogged I sucked the syrupy orange-flavoured goop into my mouth. Gels are hard work at the best of times, but this one tasted pretty good against all the seawater in my mouth. I'd clearly swallowed a lot of it as I let out a rip-roaring burp as I ran back into the sea to start my second lap.

I settled more quickly this time with fewer people around me. I knew it was just a case of concentrating and relaxing as much as possible while maintaining my pace. The first buoy came quickly and without the traffic jams, and I swam directly around it without wasting any time at all. The swell was noticeably worse on this second lap and it was difficult to see the next buoy or indeed anything at all over the height of the waves. The volunteer lifeguards were really useful, on their surfboards marking the course and keeping an eye on everybody. I could use them to help me see if the swell was too much.

As I neared the halfway point on the second lap, I felt a bit of cramp coming on in one of my calves. I'd had this before and it was no big worry at this stage. I stopped and rolled on to my back for a few seconds to stretch it out. The swell was bobbing me violently this far out in the bay and I suddenly felt overwhelmingly seasick as I stretched my legs beneath me. I took a deep breath and tried to relax but within seconds a huge jet of vomit was fountaining out of my mouth into the water in front of me. I spluttered and gagged as a second, equally violent spout flew across the water. I swam backwards trying to get away from the floating pile of rice pudding I was now bobbing around in and pulled off my nose plug to clear what felt like another gallon of rice pudding stuck in my burning nostrils.

I was shocked by how quickly I had gone from feeling completely in control into a blubbering, cramping mess. I looked around me and tried to get back some composure. In that moment I asked myself what I was going to do. It was unthinkable that I was going to quit on the swim so I had some stern words with myself. Rinsing my mouth with diesel-tainted seawater and still gagging, I got on with swimming away from the creamy slick that I had left for the poor sods behind me to swim through.

Head down and regaining composure, I was relieved to find that I was still swimming strongly and, as I rounded the last buoy for home, I knew that I was going to make it. The beach didn't come any quicker the second time around but I wasn't worried and paced myself all the way in. As I rose from the water and snot-shot the last of the rice pudding into the sand, I glanced at my watch and saw a time of one hour 47 minutes. It had been my perfect swim, and as I jogged up the zigzag to find my bag and trainers the only thing I needed to be concerned about was replacing the 500-calorie breakfast I had just left behind for the fish.

I grabbed my bag and made my way to a bench, which I knew was just a bit further up the slope. I pulled the top half of my wetsuit down to my waist and sat down to quickly wash the sand off my feet. I exchanged a few expletives with the guy next to me about the sea conditions as I pulled on my trainers and took a big bite of my banana, before carrying on up the slope into the town.

Now was definitely not the time to be raising the heart rate and burning unnecessary energy, so I jogged gently and headed through the crowds back towards the transition. The whole route was packed with faces all calling out and congratulating us and wishing us luck. It felt great and I took the time to wave to people and thank them. I saw my parents for the first time that day on a corner and waved for a photo as they cheered me by. I was in the zone and feeling good again.

As I approached the transition area, Maria, Luigi and all our other friends were cheering loudly. I gave them a clap and a smile as I went through into the transition tent and grabbed my bike bag from the rack. I found a seat and quickly towelled myself down and peeled off my wetsuit. I took my time to wash and wipe my feet of all the sand and squirted a big glug of chamois crème down the front of my tri suit. I wasn't going to be winning a place on the podium or qualifying for the Ironman World Championships today, so it was more important to take my time, be methodical and get comfortable for the rest of the day rather than rush through and forget something.

I was now dressed and ready to get on the bike, but I took a few more seconds to sit back and finish my banana and drink some water amongst all the frantic activity in the tent. I then took a deep breath, stood up, handed my bag to one of the helpers and clip-clopped out of the tent in my cycling shoes to grab my bike. Now that the worry of my worst discipline was out of the way, the next eight hours or so on the bike would be the most critical and the place where my race could really start to unravel.

Bike

THE WEATHER wasn't particularly cold for a mid-September morning in the depths of Wales, but I shivered hard as I trotted out to find my bike. Approaching two hours submerged in 16-degree water had taken its toll on my core temperature, despite my best attempts to warm up the inside of my wetsuit. I knew this was likely to happen, so despite seeing other people whizzing past me in only their tri suits and helmets, I erred on the side of caution and wore a cycle jersey, windproof gilet and arm warmers. I knew how brutally the weather can change in this part of the world, and, considering I was going to be spending eight hours or so sat on my bike, I wasn't taking any chances.

I found my bike quickly and trotted back towards the exit, pushing it out in front of me. I had already clipped my Garmin into its cradle on the handlebars and knew exactly what numbers I needed to hit to make that eight-hour bike leg a reality. Considering the pro-racers will be finishing in under five hours, eight seemed like an eternity to get it done, but this is a long-distance triathlon and you still need to average around 14 miles an hour throughout – no mean feat on a hilly course like Wales. I did the sums in my head again as I wheeled my bike to the gate.

My swim was one hour 47 plus the transition, making it roughly two hours as I crossed the line for the bike start, and eight hours on the bike would see me coming back in at the ten-hour mark, giving me about 30 minutes' grace before the cut-off. Shit that's not a lot, it only equates to about two punctures. I had played these sums over and over in my head in the days before the race and they were still just as tight and a little scary. I had to trust in my training, which was telling me I could manage it.

'Keep an eye on the numbers on the watch, pace yourself and don't linger at the aid stations,' were the words going around in my head as I crossed the line at the exit to the transition area. I swung my leg over the bike and clipped in to a big cheer from my little band of supporters. I gave them a big smile and a salute as I passed by and then slowly wound up my legs, feeling the resistance build as I clicked through the gears on my way out into the narrow streets of the town.

I glided past the last of the swimmers who were still making their way back to the transition. If they had taken the full two hours 20 minutes on their swim, plus the transition time, then they had better be decent cyclists because the timings were going to be even tighter for them. For the first time I felt like I was in a comfortable position and vowed to keep that feeling going.

I had to fuel, that was clear after my little incident in the sea, so I finished a bottle of energy drink and a gel as I settled in on my way out of town and on to the open road. I found a decent pace I knew I could maintain without pushing too hard and made my first proper inventory of the day – how was I feeling?

My legs felt fine with no weakness to speak of, and I wasn't feeling that general lethargy that struck me after the Wales Triathlon swim, so that was good. I felt a little sick but had expected that considering how much seawater I must have consumed. I was confident that the sickness would settle as the race went on and at least I wasn't going to get cramp with all that extra salt I'd consumed. The sun was now peeking through the clouds and the weather seemed to be improving all the time, and best of all there appeared to be no strong winds to speak of.

The first section out to Pembrokeshire is surprisingly hilly, but it also has some long descents to make up time, and I figured that anything over 20 miles per hour was good, so I told myself not to be reckless or push my heart rate too high in the early stages trying to chase too much speed. I also had to rein in my desire to hunt down other people who were ahead of me – I was near the back of the field and had to accept that. I was only in a race with myself today and my plan certainly didn't allow for any heroics, that was for sure. I pulled a gel from my crossbar bag and squeezed it into my mouth: 100 calories every 20 minutes, don't forget it.

Fairly soon I was shooting around the back of Pembroke and up the first of the long, steep climbs out towards the coast. As I reached the top, I heard a foreign accent calling out to me from behind. As he came alongside he asked if he could borrow my pump as he had already suffered a puncture and he couldn't get enough air into his tyre with his. I was making good time, so we pulled over and he got to work pumping away frantically with my little race pump. He was Norwegian and had travelled over especially for the race.

After about three minutes he thanked me profusely and off he went, and I mounted up and followed suit only to see him disappear quickly into the distance ahead of me. I was pleased to have helped someone out, as I would hope that someone might do the same for me, but in a sickening wave of realisation it was clear that he could afford to spend a few minutes at the roadside. I, on the other hand, wasn't in such a luxurious position and had just taken a big bite out of one of my two puncture stops. I knew that there was no way I could be doing that again.

A tight, gravelly and wet descent through some trees saw a few brave or stupid people flying past me but I wasn't compromising on my 'safety first, speed second' rule, so I let them go. I could tell by my heart rate monitor that I was still in the safe zone as I inched back past them on the next climb. All the climbing I had done in training was allowing me to ride a much steadier and more controlled race than some of the other maybe less well-trained back markers around me.

I knew the course like the back of my hand and exactly where I could use my tri bars to full effect; getting into a tuck gave me at least half a mile an hour extra for no more effort and I was smoothly rolling out some of these sections at 19 or 20 miles an hour, well over the average I would need to maintain for the course. I flew through the beach sections at Freshwater West and Angle and was back again on the long drag towards Pembroke. This was where your average speed can get a real boost, but I made a crucial decision not to go all out, and although I could have worked harder to make up more time I reserved some energy and tucked in at a steady pace. I remembered how I flew through this section on the Long Course Weekend and paid horribly for it later when the real hills started.

A long line of colourful cyclists rolled into Pembroke as the course took itself all the way down the high street and back in front of the crowds of spectators all cheering encouragement and well wishes. I had my first wobble at the end of the high street as a complete U-turn was needed around a traffic cone in front of lots of pairs of watching eyes – certainly not the time to be having a low-speed fall – and, despite my pretty mediocre bike handling skills, I successfully wobbled around it in one piece and headed out of town towards the first of the aid stations.

If one thing was playing on my mind it was the fact that I hadn't yet been to the toilet and familiar rumblings and cramping sensations were now starting to twinge inside me. It was good timing as I was approaching the first of the aid stations where I knew there would be some Portaloos. I decided to burn some more of my precious puncture repair time and make a stop that, fingers crossed, would pay off for the rest of the day. Hopefully the toilets would also be in a reasonable condition this early in the race.

As I pulled up into the village hall car park and slipped off my bike, my legs were already beginning to buckle a bit under me as I tottered off towards the toilets and stepped into an unoccupied cubicle. It was clean enough; I could deal with the piss all over the seat and it even had a roll of toilet paper hanging from a chain above the door. I had decided to wear my tri suit throughout the day but this meant I had to strip off a lot of layers to get out of it. The gilet came off first, followed by my cycle jersey and then I could slip my shoulders out of my tri suit and pull it down, leaving me virtually naked as I sat down. After what then felt like a lifetime, I let out a long, low-pitched fart which rattled around in the little plastic box I was crouched in, and then that was it. I sat for a little while longer waiting and waiting as slowly but surely the panicking started. I couldn't sit there all bloody day, and after such a work-up I now knew damned well that nothing was going to be happening anytime soon. I got up and started to redress in a hurry and swore out loud as I put the wrong arm in my cycle jersey and wrestled around in the rocking Portaloo trying to get back out as quickly as I could. Every second I was stuck in that box felt like a minute and when I eventually sprang back out of the door I was another precious few minutes down.

That aid station signals the start of the so-called 'hilly bit' of the course and it introduces itself with a long steady climb right from the off. Like all of that bloody course, I knew that hill very well and as the people around me got out of their saddles and pumped themselves into their red zones I sat back and eased myself up. There was a farmhouse on the left about halfway up and I knew that the climb eased off slightly after that. I reached it and knocked down a couple of gears, and keeping the same steady effort I reeled back in most of those who had whizzed ahead and were now struggling to reach the top.

These little tactical choices helped my confidence no end, but what was a little disconcerting was the fact that the professional and elite racers were one by one already passing me on their second laps. They flew past like I was standing still and it was a truly mind-blowing sight to behold. As a crumb of consolation I told myself that they probably hadn't been subjected to the 'Mother of all Surgery' only a few months before and I knuckled down to the job at hand, which just happened to be grinding out another 70-odd miles.

The crowds were unbelievable around the whole course. In the small towns and villages the streets were lined with people as the bunting flapped in the wind and the air was filled with applause. Even out into the countryside, families who were trapped at home by the closed roads were having barbecues and parties in their front gardens to join in with the celebrations. I passed a tractor in an entrance to a field with an old sofa slung high up in its scoop, and a whole family seemed to be squashed on to it watching the race.

The sun was now shining brightly from between the clouds and the weather was warming up nicely. I had shed the gilet and was feeling comfortable as we glided past the pebble beach and a beautiful shimmering sea at

Wiseman's Bridge. There were a lot of the faster riders passing me now and the course was quite congested as we rolled towards the first of the two big coastal climbs. Once again I settled into my highest gear right at the bottom and let people come past me until they hit the steep section through the woods. This was a tough climb and my legs were like lead by the time I got to the top, but it was negotiated smoothly, leaving quite a few wobbling in my wake as I sailed over the top and down into the next bay.

This is probably the most dangerous descent of the whole course and is always damp and gravelly with an adverse camber on the tightest of the bends near the bottom where you have picked up the most speed. As I rounded the corner I grabbed a handful of brake just as my back wheel lost grip on the gravel. The wheel, along with my backside, twitched violently and I wrestled to regain control of my bike as I swept around the curve and was spat out at the bottom. So much for keeping my heart rate out of the red, that was a proper close shave. I made a note to take more care on the second lap.

I was now in the centre of Saundersfoot riding towards the foot of Heartbreak Hill, the showpiece of the whole cycle race where the biggest crowds gathered. They spill on to the road and then part like the sea as the athletes struggle through them on the steepest sections. For one brief moment you are in the Tour de France and if you were going to put on a bit of a show, then this was the time to be doing it. I stood up out of my saddle for the first time in the race and powered through the crowds to unbelievable cheering, and I even got a couple of pats on the back as the sea of bodies parted and I passed through. When I popped out of the crowds, I was blowing hard and my heart rate was way too high but the buzz from it was great and I managed to channel that feeling all the way to the top of that long climb. Before I knew it, I was turning out the big gears and whizzing my way back to Tenby.

I took a moment to call out for my special-needs bag, which was passed to me on the move like a pro-racer, and I stuffed the gels and flapjacks I had in it into my pouch ready for the second lap. I delved in again, as there was a secret weapon inside that I had been looking forward to for a while. Triumphantly I pulled out a cheese and Marmite roll before discarding the bag with one of the volunteers. I unwrapped it as I rolled along and took a big bite. Its salty goodness was awesome but it instantly stuck to the roof of my dry mouth like concrete and I had to swill it down with some orange energy drink. It took away some of the joy but it still gave me the big salty carbohydrate boost that my body was craving.

The bike course rolled down into town alongside the run course and already there were people out on it. How I wished at that stage that I could have joined them, but I still had about 45 miles of cycling to get out of the way. As I flew down into the bottom of town, some cyclists were peeling off to the left and heading towards the transition, but I was turning right through the barriers and heading back out of town on to the open road again, and as I swung right at full speed I heard loud cheers and my name being called out.

I turned to see my supporters all waving and cheering me through, and I waved back and got lost in the moment for a second too long. When I turned back to the road I was alarmed to see that I had drifted right and was now dangerously close to the legs of the barriers. I swerved back out into the road with my heart in my mouth. Fucking hell! I berated myself as this was the second close call I had dodged in a very short space of time. I knew I was getting tired, but I had to concentrate or I could lose everything and it would be my own stupid fault.

The cyclists had noticeably thinned out around me as I headed out on my second lap, and this is where I really needed to knuckle down to business and not let up on the pace. My addled brain was constantly going over the sums in my head, and although I believed I was still good for time one thing was clear: with the stops I hadn't made up any time on that first lap and it was still going to be a tight finish.

As the hills rolled by the quiet concentration of everyone left on the course was palpable. The 'no drafting' rule meant that we had to stay at least ten metres behind each other and overtake quickly so there was little opportunity to chat. On the hills, people bunched together more as they tried to overtake and there was time for a few words of encouragement and some banter to lighten the mood and take our minds off of the exhaustion for a few moments. You couldn't linger too long though, as the motorcycle judges were constantly on the prowl and always keeping a beady eye on us.

All this quiet time slogging along in your own miserable little bubble plays havoc with your mind. I constantly had panics where I convinced myself I wasn't going to make it back in time as I'd made a catastrophic miscalculation in pace. These were followed by long periods of frantic Einstein-sized equations going around in my head before I could convince myself I was still safe, only to go through the same painful process all over again a few minutes later.

The constant mental arithmetic was now starting to become more exhausting than the cycling, and trust me the cycling was truly exhausting. My lower back was really starting to ache where my weak abdominal muscles didn't have the strength to support it and, although my legs were still spinning, my thighs were burning with lactic acid and my backside was becoming numb due to the thin padding of my tri suit, and to cap it all my face was still throbbing painfully from that bloody jellyfish sting.

After what seemed like an age and my average speed dropping like a stone with each subsequent climb, I was back at Wiseman's Bridge for the big effort through the trees again. This time the scene I was confronted with was one of utter devastation, cyclists weaving wildly from left to right, some stopped at the side of the road with their limbs poking out at ridiculous angles as they desperately tried to stretch off cramps. One guy I rolled slowly past was sobbing as he gripped his thigh in agony. I was again in danger of being knocked off, so I picked my route carefully and crawled past the carnage and surfaced at the top in one piece.

Rolling more gently down that treacherous descent, I knew I could start to relax a bit when I got to the bottom, as with only one big hill left to climb I would be on my way back into the transition. Barring a crash or a mechanical failure, I was home and dry, and with every pedal stroke my confidence grew as I was yet another metre closer to home, meaning I would be more able to run in with the bike on my shoulder if it came to it.

Back at Heartbreak Hill, I didn't get the same boost I had received the first time around – although there were still a few hardy souls cheering us on, the big crowds had long since buggered off to the pub. I pumped my lonely way up to a few cheers at the top and before I knew it I was freewheeling quickly back towards town and the transition.

The run course was now packed with athletes as the last of us weary souls rolled our way past them. The winners had by now already finished and were probably showered and already celebrating. One last nasty little hill couldn't take the shine off the relief of hitting the town proper, and as I rolled back into the transition with a couple of other smiling athletes, we congratulated each other and wished each other luck for the rest of the day. I slowed as I approached the dismount line and saw Maria, my parents and friends all at the barrier smiling and clapping. The relief on their faces was obvious. I gave them another big salute and with a broad smile swung my leg over my bike to get off. It nearly buckled under me as it touched the ground. My legs were certainly going to take a while to adjust as I swaggered over the line like John Wayne and racked my bike back in its place in the now packed transition area. I patted it on the saddle and thanked it for looking after me all day as it had performed immaculately.

I had crossed the line in eight hours and 47 seconds, exactly what I said I would do. It gave me a race time of ten hours and four minutes, only 26 minutes before the cut-off. But now that I was back in, that didn't matter for shit and I was elated. It was part sheer relief for being able to get off that bloody bike at last and part exhausted hysteria for having made it back at all.

I hobbled into the transition tent, grabbed my transition bag and slumped heavily into a chair. I took a moment to fish out a banana and look around as I took a bite. The scene in that tent was a desperate one – a lot of people had clearly turned themselves inside out to make the cut and were now in a terrible state trying to get themselves together before they got back out on the run course. People were lying half-naked on the ground trying to stretch out their seized-up backs, while others seemed to be wandering around in a daze. Sat down a few seats from me was a man with his head in his hands gently sobbing his heart out, and he wasn't the only one crying, either – there were a lot of overwhelmed people in that tent.

I stooped to peel off my socks and change into my running trainers. I pulled off my sweaty cycling jersey and pulled on my running visor. My tri suit was crusted with sweat and a dollop of chamois cream was squirted down the front of it on to my shrivelled bits and another big dollop smeared across my nipples. I reset my watch and calculated that I had just shy of seven hours to complete the marathon. There was only one more cut-off to hit and that was in about six hours' time with about ten kilometres left to race – it was eminently doable. I finished my banana and took a big confident swig from my water bottle. I didn't want to linger, so I forced myself to get creakily up from the chair and to get moving, stepping over the bodies as I went.

As I exited the tent and walked towards the exit I wondered in my head when exactly I needed to start running. The answer was of course as soon as I liked or even better right there and then, but my body seemed physically unable to fire the right nerves in the right order to make it happen. I knew that once I started I wasn't going to stop until I'd either collapsed or hit that finish line, and my body was desperately trying to tell me that it would be a much better idea just to stop and lie down. My body may not have wanted it but mentally I was still pushing forwards, and this race was now all in my hands or, more accurately, my feet. No mechanical failures could stop me now and if it came to it I could crawl towards the line. After all, I only had a marathon left to run.

Run

THE FAN club was outside, so it was time to impress again. I gingerly put one foot in front of the other and wound myself up into a gentle trot. The legs screamed and wobbled but they were still working, and before I knew it I was half-stumbling, half-jogging out under the arch as the last of the bike finishers were being ushered quickly over the line with just seconds to spare. Some had an agonising wait to see if they could continue while the stewards checked their chip times against the gun time, and some didn't make the cut by just a few agonising seconds and, head in hands, were being led away.

A big cheer greeted me as I appeared and it sent me on my way, and with a big smile I waved and called out, asking where Tom was. Maria shouted back that he was about 15 minutes ahead of me. I was so relieved to hear that he had made it in off the bike and, like me, it was all now in his hands. I turned away as I was starting to well up again. I suddenly felt overwhelmed by the fantastic support I was receiving; every one of them was willing me on but in that moment I felt so weak and undeserving of all the support and belief pouring my way. I was desperate not to let anyone down but as I got into my stride the painful truth was dawning on me just how crushingly tired I was.

I would still have to run most of the marathon to get it done within the time limit and in that first kilometre it was clear that it was mind over matter that was going to get me there. My body was crying out to stop and walk as I skirted the medieval town walls and out on to the course proper. The run course is not barricaded off from the crowds like the rest of the race and it was surreal to be having to dodge people licking ice creams and gawping as I went by, and some seemed to be doing their level best to get in my way or trip me up.

I kept the legs turning and jogged my way out of town aided by a decent descent which took me on to the open roads. Like all multi-lap races, midway through each lap you receive a coloured arm band which shows how many of the four laps you have completed. It was here, as I observed the other runners, that I had my first bout of a phenomenon known as band envy – seeing those with even one more band than me meant they had at least ten kilometres less than me left to run. If I had the energy to lynch one of them for even one of those bands, I think I would have done it.

At least half of the run is uphill and the first ascent started right away, ramping up alarmingly ahead of me. My pace slowed instantly to a walk as I hit the incline and I was frustrated by the lack of power I was able to put out. I couldn't walk the whole course and on this first lap I needed to get a decent ten-kilometre time in the bag, so mustering everything I had I started to run again. Taking baby steps, I gritted my teeth and trotted my way through the steepest section towards the first aid station.

Each subsequent aid station after that became like a little oasis for me. I told myself I could walk while I took on my fuel and this little treat then propelled me forwards towards the next aid station where I could treat myself again. This deal was well and truly sealed when at that first aid station I took a cup of water and a cup of flat cola. When that cola touched my lips it was like fireworks going off in my mouth. The taste of it was like nectar after the bland fake fruit flavours I had been enduring all day and I lurched on with the thought of the next delicious little cup driving me forwards.

I ran all of that first lap and collected my first band on the turn. Pulling it on to my arm was a big boost which helped propel me back down the hill towards the town. The course took a cruel little uphill dog-leg around another lonely traffic cone and a timing mat to ensure no one 'forgot' to do it and then headed towards the crowded, narrow streets of Tenby. We rounded the harbour, where we had completed the swim what now felt like days before, and turned right to head up into the high street. As I turned the corner, my exhausted brain raced as I tried to compute what I was seeing in front of me.

Under flapping bunting strung everywhere was a sea of heads stretching out for the entire length of the high street. A wall of noise hit me like a tidal wave, hundreds of partying people all cheering at once. Down the middle of this drunken ocean weaved a thin band of tarmac through which a line of stooping athletes ran or shuffled. As I moved forwards through it, I started to feel giddy and overwhelmed. I was engulfed by the crowd as people leant in towards me pumping their fists and calling out my name as they read it from my race number. They were passionately encouraging me to dig deep and push harder and I flinched and almost tripped as my head spun with it all. The high street kicked cruelly upwards and my body was screaming out for me to walk, but how could I amongst all that support? I pushed on, turning my exhausted legs ever forwards, and just stared at the ground. I could feel the tears coming again.

I told myself I could walk when I broke through the top of the crowd, but with every turn there were more and more people within touching distance exalting me to keep going, so I kept going. I spotted my little supporters' club ahead of me in the crowd on one of the narrowest streets. Bugger it! I can't walk now. They saw me coming and the cheer was the loudest of the day. I high-fived them as I jogged past. Luigi looked me in the eye and shouted, 'You've got this.' At that point I was feeling anything but, the only thing I'd got was a bit over-emotional.

A cruel twist of the course meant that as you popped out through a medieval gateway in the old town wall it either turned left on to the Esplanade and the last 400 metres to the red carpet and the promised land of the finish line, or turned right and out for another long painful lap. As you passed through the arch you could hear the music pumping and the crowds at the finish, which was tantalisingly close but still so very far away. I still had to make that agonising right turn two more times before I could turn left.

The second lap went past in a blur. I ran when I could but found myself increasingly walking on the hills. The cola at the aid stations was all that seemed to be leapfrogging me between them. I didn't see Tom on the course that lap and prayed that he was still going. As I approached town for the second time I felt the wind picking up. I was starting to get dark and light rain was swirling in the blustery light of the street lamps, which one by one were slowly beginning to flicker on. The course was also getting noticeably lonelier as the majority of the athletes now streaming under the arch were making that left turn.

I wasn't moving fast enough to keep my heart rate or my body temperature up now and dressed in just my tri suit I was starting to feel cold, very cold. I called out to Maria that I would need a long-sleeve jersey on the next lap and she agreed to meet me with it at the special needs area. I also made a diva-like request for some roast chicken for when I was finished, just to keep her on her toes that late in the evening and give me something to look forward to.

I saw my parents loom out of the darkness on a quieter part of the course and walked alongside them as they asked me how I was feeling. I could see in my mum's eyes that she was getting worried about me. I was now feeling cold, weak and a little disorientated. I couldn't waste energy chatting so I turned and jogged away from them. I was surprised how lonely I was feeling now that it was dark, despite the support which was still all over the course.

I kept going, running on the flats and down hills and power walking the ups. It was now quicker for me and less painful to walk the ups than try to run them. I had two bands on my arm and was heading towards my third, so I was slowly but surely getting it done. On the bike I was constantly calculating my times but I was now far too exhausted to cope with anything other than concentrating on putting one foot in front of the other. I was still in the depths of the race at this stage and wasn't convinced that I had it in the bag as I plodded along.

Half done and now only a half-marathon to go. The numbers didn't matter anymore, all that mattered was continuing to move forwards, but this was getting harder and harder to do. I swore under my breath as I started to slow to a walk even on some of the flats. This was where my race was starting to unravel. I was starting to feel sorry for myself and with my battered body now soaked by the drizzly rain the cold was really starting to take its toll – even the magical colas were starting to make me gag.

It was as I walked with my drinks at one of the mid-course aid stations I fell in alongside another runner who was limping as he made his way into the darkness. We got talking and it turned out he was a firefighter, and as a copper we had a bit of blue-light affinity, so walked and talked about the race and where we worked. It felt good to have some company and a few jokes lifted my mood and helped take my mind off the pain for a while. It transpired that his hip was in agony from an old injury and he didn't think he could run much more. I was happy at that stage to drop in and speed walk with him as it gave me a chance not to have to run for a bit and I needed the excuse.

I had just finished my cola and a water when a hot flush came over me, my stomach suddenly felt like it had turned to stone and waves of cramping rolled around my guts. I physically couldn't keep going so I stopped, put my hands on my knees and vomited on to the road ahead of me. What seemed like gallons of steaming flat cola and water splashed on to the wet tarmac and my trainers before running like a river between my legs back down the hill. Three long retches later I was feeling a little light-headed but much better. I shook my head and as my mind cleared I realised what a daze I had been in for at least the last hour or so. I suddenly felt like I was back in the game.

My digestive system had finally surrendered and pulled down the shutters after 14-odd hours, so I was going to have to rely on what dwindling supplies of energy I had left inside me to get around. I caught back up with my new best mate Dave the fireman and we disappeared off into the night. At the furthest turn on the course Tom suddenly lurched like a zombie out of the darkness towards us. He was probably only about ten minutes ahead of me now and had slowed down massively. He looked terrible but I was chuffed to pieces that I'd spotted him and he was still alive and, more importantly, still moving forwards. He urged me to catch him up, but unless he was lying flat out on the road taking a nap, I knew it was going to be highly unlikely.

Dave and I managed to run for a bit down from the turn and walked through the checkpoint to collect our third arm bands. We discussed the times and between both of our exhausted brains we managed to work out that we were going to make it if we kept moving. It was surreal to think that in a couple of hours' time I could actually be an Ironman. It was so dark and cold out on the course that you would be hard-pressed not to think that the whole thing was already finished and everyone had gone home and not told us.

As we walked back into town, the high street had been deserted by the big crowds of earlier but there were still a few drunkards lurching about to chase us up the road. We ran sporadically when we were encouraged to do so and before we knew it we were turning right for the last time. Looking left, we couldn't see it around the corner, but could tell that the Esplanade was lit up by the bright lights and the pumping music of the finish line. We had about two and a half hours to cover the last ten kilometres and then we could see it for ourselves.

The volunteers at the checkpoint congratulated us and clapped us on our way as we collected our fourth and final arm bands with broad smiles. I told Dave I wanted to run for a bit but he said he was in too much pain so I stuck with him and we power walked back towards town. I knew I had a little left to give so was determined to run it in if I could.

As we got to the outskirts of town we were shocked to see someone lying at the side of the road being tended to by some members of the public who had probably been walking home. The poor sod only had about a mile and a half to go. I strained my eyesight into the gloom to make sure it wasn't Tom. It wasn't, but even at this late stage it was sobering to think that anything could still happen.

As we hit town for the last time, the wind was blowing us sideways and the rain was really coming down, but the well wishes of the few hardy souls who were still around helped to warm us up. The cheers of encouragement had now been replaced with shouts of congratulations. We now had probably less than half a mile to go and over an hour to get it done. I was going to make it, I was going to be an Ironman.

A sudden rush of blood got me running through the town again and although Dave was complaining bitterly he came along with me. We snaked around the last few streets being clapped all the way and before we knew it we were at the arch and could at last make that magical left turn. Stood right in front of me crying her eyes out and jumping up and down was Maria. I shook Dave's hand and told him to enjoy it. He disappeared around the corner into the light and I went straight across the road and fell into Maria's arms.

I was so proud of her for supporting me through that last year and this win was as much for her as it was for me. I was so pleased I was going to bring it home for her. She told me to go and enjoy it and I peeled away and ran out on to the Esplanade into a flood of light and on towards the pumping music. The red carpet stretched out in front of me and at the end of it was the Ironman finishing line. The route either side was packed with people.

As I ran towards the light I saw my parents at the barrier. My mum squealed with delight as I ran over and hugged her tight. I shook my dad's hand and he patted me on the back. It was a perfect end seeing them there just before the finish. I'm sure they thought I was mad when I said I was going to attempt it and I could see how proud they were. I knew that as my parents they must have felt every inch of the pain I had suffered that year and by finishing this race I could show them that I was still fighting hard.

It was now the moment for me to celebrate and as I ran towards the red carpet I felt like I was floating on air. All the pain and exhaustion of the last 16 hours dropped away as the cheers got louder and louder, lifting me higher and higher. As I took my first steps on to the red carpet I weaved from side to side, showboating and high-fiving the crowd each side of the runway as the finish got closer and closer. Then I heard the words I'd wanted to hear for so long.

'PAUL, YOU ARE AN IRONMAN!'

As I crossed the line I leapt up and punched the air, I roared out loud as ten months of pent-up fear and uncertainty was released all at once. As I came back down my legs buckled under me and I almost fell as I staggered forwards. My head was in a spin as I shook hands with the dignitaries and a medal was hung around my neck. I looked down at it and pressed it hard to my chest – it was one of the best things I had seen in my whole life.

I looked up and there was Tom waiting for me with a big smile on his exhausted face. We embraced and congratulated each other. Neither of us could quite believe it.

I had only gone and bloody done it. I was an Ironman.

Epilogue

IT IS now approaching three years since I crossed the finish line in a time of 16 hours, five minutes and 24 seconds on that wet and windy night in Wales and, although those years have thankfully been cancer-free, I can't say my life has been entirely free from medical incident. Just 18 months after the race I found myself back on a drip sniffing those familiar warm smells of the bowel ward while covering everything in fountains of green vomit as another NG tube was forced down the wrong nostril.

That week in hospital with a painful bowel obstruction caused by scar tissue strangling my insides did wonders for correcting the upwardly creeping numbers on the bathroom scales, but it also reminded me that my life looks very different now than it did before my brush with the 'Mother of all Surgery'. After such an invasive operation there are always adjustments to be made, and I have to be careful to stay hydrated and I still get bouts of bowel pain which can often linger for weeks at a time. I still get caught short more often than most and at all the worst times, but on the whole I live a healthy and happy life free from the worry of cancer. It probably wouldn't be a good idea for me to go on a jungle trek or an arctic expedition anytime soon because of the risks, but if I did I'm pretty sure the travel insurance premiums would prove to be far more painful than falling ill.

My life has been affected in so many ways since I had that crazy idea to do an Ironman. When I first considered the possibility that I could get my chubby body around a course like that there was no fucking way in a million years it was going to happen. People loved the sentiment but did anyone really think I could manage it? Probably not in private, but openly I found so much positivity in the people around me that it spurred me on.

Setting such a long-term goal required persistence and organisation on a previously unheard of level. I had to shed those lazy Sundays lingering in my pyjamas till lunchtime and get my arse out of the door in the wind and rain to get those long sessions done. I had to give up pressing the snooze button on my alarm clock until Maria shouted at me to get up, and actually get up to go for that swim at six in the morning. Before that I don't think I had ever done anything before six in the morning, let alone go for a swim.

Ah! Swimming, my least favourite, favourite sport. What the hell was I thinking? I hated the swimming. I still hate swimming but at least now I can do it. Why on earth didn't I just do an ultra-marathon? The nearest I would have got to water would have been a muddy puddle. The reason isn't entirely clear to me, but I think deep down that I was trying to define what a real challenge meant to me. A marathon is a challenge but so was the first half-marathon I did, and wasn't my first ten-kilometre run a challenge at the time? Of course they were, but they were all eminently doable. A challenge should be defined as something that there is a real possibility of failing. I had to ask the questions of myself that at least matched the ones being asked by the cancer.

Focussing the mind was the key for me to get through the whole experience. Cancer can easily overwhelm your thoughts and forcing my head to share its space with something that is equally as much of a head fuck as cancer did wonders for watering down the negative thoughts that creep around. Crippling tiredness is also a big plus, because when you can't keep your eyes open past eight in the evening, it ensures that you're not lying awake in bed all night thinking negative thoughts.

The other big bonus I got from it all was the positive progress I made pretty much from the moment I woke up in intensive care right up to the finish line. Always focussing on the small gains either in physical sporting achievements or simply going a day without shitting my pants all added up to make my life a positive forward-moving adventure as opposed to being paralysed by the fear of the cancer.

The activity I was doing worked wonders for my physical recovery. I believe wholeheartedly that by training as hard as I did it mobilised and softened the scar tissue and got my body back to health far quicker and to a greater level than if I had taken it easy worrying about hernias and feeling sorry for myself. I now reap those rewards by being back doing all the sports and activities I enjoyed before the operation and all relatively pain-free.

It's been said that anyone can do an Ironman and you know what? It's bloody well true. If I could manage it after what I went through then so can you. Consider the thought of it for a moment. Fucking ridiculous, you say. Wait a minute, didn't you hear me say that? The reality is that every part of that race can be broken down and worked on, small progressions lead to the biggest prizes. That's true of anything in life – you can build a plan, stick to it and you will get there eventually. There is not one type of body at the Ironman, trust me I've seen some real sights in those transition tents. All ages and all shapes and sizes achieve that dream, they just dream bigger than most, so why can't you do that? You really can.

Do I regret the diagnosis or any of the experiences I have been through? As strange as it may sound I wouldn't change a single thing about my life. The last few years have been incredibly hard and painful at times but they have shaped me into who I am today. I am slimmer, fitter and with a bigger lust for adventure and new experiences than I ever had before.

I took my life for granted. My marriage to Maria, which was always good, has been strengthened enormously by my absolute respect for her. The overwhelming love and support she has shown me since day one has made me understand our relationship on a much deeper level and has brought me even closer to her. She couldn't get rid of me now even if she wanted to – not even the cancer was able to do that.

My relationships with my friends have also deepened. Good friends are hard to find and I have always counted them on one hand. Since I've had to face up to the fact that we may not be around for each other forever, I value and treasure the time I spend with them so much more.

Would I trade the risk of the cancer returning for losing my new outlook on life? The simple answer is no, because I could still be run over by that bus tomorrow. The fragility of life hasn't changed, so why should I? This whole journey has given me the privilege of seeing life through a brand new lens and I now see so much more because of it.

My feelings on what it means to have cancer have also changed after having to deal with it. When I was diagnosed I was all 'fuck you cancer', but that view has softened. The reality is that cancer is a mutation of our own cells and not a foreign invader. When you say 'fuck cancer' you are saying 'fuck off' to your own body. The cold truth is that you either get better with the best medicine and treatments available to you or you don't – you have little say in the proceedings other than your willingness to fight. The sentiment 'I will fight this' is, however, very different. It's a natural human instinct to fight for your life, but no one with a terminal diagnosis should be made to feel that they could have beaten it if only they had fought harder. It just doesn't work like that, you cannot physically fight the cancer, the doctors do that bit. What you can do is prepare the body and mind that surrounds the cancer to make it ready for that fight, and for me it was with fitness.

I'm not one for dishing out advice but reflecting on my experiences if I had to give some it would be to enjoy your life to the full and be as healthy and happy as you can be right now, not to leave it until you get a kick up the arse from a health scare. If you are in poor health you will only have a much bigger mountain to climb when you are trying to recover. If that means doing a triathlon, obstacle race or a five-kilometre parkrun then so be it, but it could just as easily be going for a long walk and getting some fresh air in your lungs.

In a world where there are no guarantees, the one thing that is guaranteed for me is that I now go to tackle my annual cancer scans as an Ironman. If the cancer returns, I will fight again and this time I'll be fitter and stronger still and, while doing so, I will keep on enjoying everything that life has to offer me. The Ironman motto is, 'anything is possible', and as I ran up that red carpet I discovered that it really is true. I only have to glance down at my Ironman tattoo to remind me of that.

Acknowledgements

MY WIFE Maria, whose unwavering love, support and belief from that first sunny day in August 2014 to now has allowed me to achieve all the things I could only previously have dreamed of.

My good friend Tom, whose bloody stupid idea it was in the first place, and whom I had the pleasure of beating by one whole minute.

Mr Faheez Mohamed and Mr Sanjeev Dayal, the wonderful consultants whose expertise and knowledge of this rare disease undoubtedly saved my life.

Linda Cass and all the nurses, nursing assistants, physiotherapists and everybody else associated with ward C2 at the Basingstoke and North Hampshire Hospital. You are all angels.

The Southcote Surgery. It's easy to moan about your local doctors' surgery, but when it mattered they really came through, and without their timely intervention my outcome could have been so much worse.

Don Fink, the author of *Be Iron Fit*. Without the structure of this programme, I would never have managed my training time effectively enough. If you are considering an Ironman, give it a read.

Laura Priest, my wonderful sports massage therapist from Holistic Beauty in Reading. She made my eyes water and my aching limbs work right up to race day.

Kelly Rutledge of Rutledge Sports Therapy. Her excellent treatment kept me in the game when it really mattered.

My race day supporters' club, you all know who you are and your vocal support on the day gave me the boost I needed at all the right times.

My family who will always love and believe in me, and finally to my best friend Luigi, who always has my back when it matters.

Thank you.

If you have enjoyed reading *Dead Man to Ironman: A Ten-Month Journey from Dead Meat to Athlete* please take a moment to give it a review.

If you have any questions about Pseudomyxoma Peritonei (PMP), triathlon or anything else for that matter, I'd love to hear from you. Get in touch or spread the love at:

deadmeattoathlete.com
Deadmeattoathlete@hotmail.com
#deadmeattoathlete